AF513363

The *Body* Alarm

Dr Aakanksha Gupta brings preventive healthcare to the forefront of daily consciousness, enabling individuals and communities to take ownership of their well-being. An MBBS graduate with a postgraduate degree from IIM Calcutta and a Harvard certification in Global Health Quality and Safety, she is also a TEDx speaker, the author of *First Aid Handbook*, and a next-generation thought leader who inspires a shift towards proactive, prevention-based healthcare.

She can be reached on:

LinkedIn: https://www.linkedin.com/in/dr-aakanksha-gupta/
Instagram: https://www.instagram.com/thebodyalarm/
X: https://x.com/doctoraakanksha

'*The* body speaks long before disease appears. *The Body Alarm* sensitively reminds readers to observe these early signals and respond with awareness and responsibility. By bridging modern medical insight with the timeless wisdom of prevention, this book encourages a more conscious, balanced and sustainable approach to health for individuals and families alike.'

—Dr Partap Chauhan

Director, Jiva Ayurveda; Author of three bestselling books

'*The Body Alarm* is a timely and thoughtful contribution to preventive healthcare, translating complex clinical ideas into clear signals that students and young professionals can act upon. It encourages a culture of early diagnosis, responsibility and body-literate citizenship. Dr Gupta masterfully converts complex medical signals into essential "preventive intelligence" for today's youth. This book is a crucial addition to student welfare, making health literacy and early detection as fundamental as academic excellence. Her systematic approach to symptom recognition is precisely what young people need—transforming health literacy from reactive fear into proactive intelligence. A bold, evidence-rich framework that could genuinely save lives if widely adopted.'

—Prof. Yogesh Singh

Vice-Chancellor, University of Delhi

'*The Body Alarm* offers a powerful reminder that awareness—of the body, mind and patterns—is essential to living well. It beautifully echoes Indic wisdom, which emphasizes listening to subtle signals before imbalances turn into illness, while presenting modern medical insights aligned with dharma, responsibility and self-awareness. A meaningful contribution to holistic education and conscious living.'

—Sajjan Agarwal

Chairman and Chief Executive Officer, GreenHawk Corporation

'*The Body Alarm* beautifully reminds us that illness rarely arrives unannounced—our body always speaks before they break. With clear medical insight, relatable examples and powerful storytelling, the book empowers readers to recognize early warning signs without fear or denial.'

—Laxmi Narain Goel

Chairman, Suncity Projects

The *Body* Alarm

Simple Steps for Health and Longevity

Dr Aakanksha Gupta

RUPA

Published by
Rupa Publications India Pvt. Ltd 2026
161-B/4, Gulmohar House,
Yusuf Sarai Community Centre,
New Delhi 110049

Sales centres
Bengaluru Chennai
Hyderabad Kolkata Mumbai

Copyright © Aakanksha Gupta 2026
Illustrations courtesy: Aakanksha Gupta

The views and opinions expressed in this book are the author's own and the facts are as reported by her, which have been verified to the extent possible, and the publishers are not in any way liable for the same.

All rights reserved.
No part of this publication may be reproduced, transmitted or stored in a retrieval system, in any form or by any means, electronic, mechanical, photocopying, recording or otherwise, without the prior permission of the publisher.

P-ISBN: 978-93-5352-152-3
E-ISBN: 978-93-5352-711-2

First impression 2026

10 9 8 7 6 5 4 3 2 1

The moral right of the author has been asserted.

Printed in India

This book is sold subject to the condition that it shall not, by way of trade or otherwise, be lent, resold, hired out or otherwise circulated, without the publisher's prior consent, in any form of binding or cover other than that in which it is published.

To my lion-hearted father
Ajay Gupta

To my courageous mother
Deepshikha

and

To my forever strength,
my brother Aakash

Contents

Part 4
Pillars of Preventive Healthcare

PART 1

WHEN THE ALARM GOES UNHEARD

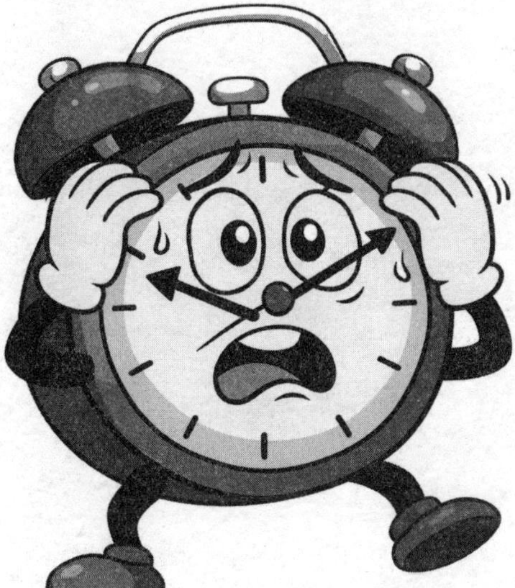

The Beautiful Chaos of Being Human

Bodies are bizarre. They gurgle, creak, twitch and do things that sound like they belong in a horror movie (for instance, random nighttime leg cramps). Most of the time, these quirks aren't just normal but hilariously normal.

Ever sneezed when you looked at the sun? That's a real reflex called the photic sneeze. Ever felt your foot cramp the second you stretched in bed? Blame your muscles for being mischievous. Ever had your stomach growl so loudly that you wondered if it was trying to communicate in Morse code? It's just digestion—no secret messages are being conveyed.

The human body is equal parts miraculous and ridiculous. It's a wonder we function at all, let alone as smoothly as we usually do.

The Limits of Knowledge

Even our most advanced science reveals more questions than answers. We still don't fully understand why some people develop chronic pain and others don't. We can't predict who will respond to which treatments. Still, we continue acting as though we are just one more supplement, one more lifestyle hack or one more diagnostic test away from the total mastery of our biology.

The Myth of Perfect Control

The pursuit of perfect control is a deeply ingrained ideal that promises safety, success and certainty in a chaotic world. However, the reality is that life's inherent unpredictability makes perfect control not only impossible but also counterproductive. This myth influences decisions, shapes behaviours and fuels stress, ultimately limiting our potential.

Nowhere is this more evident than in the realm of health. We are told that if we eat the right foods, exercise enough and avoid toxins, we can outsmart diseases. However, autoimmune conditions defy this logic. They strike without warning, even in those who did everything 'right'. The body turns against itself, and suddenly, the illusion of control shatters.

The human body is not a machine that responds predictably to inputs. Identical twins raised in the same household can develop radically different health profiles. Marathon runners suffer cardiac arrests. Lifelong smokers live to a hundred. The healthiest eater you know might be diagnosed with a serious illness tomorrow, while their fast-food-loving neighbour remains inexplicably robust.

So, as we move forward, remember: You are not a machine. You don't need perfect metrics. You don't need to panic over every blip. You just need to pay attention with curiosity, patience and maybe even a little bit of humour.

Your Body Doesn't Do 'Drama'

The human body is an ancient, finely tuned system that responds, adapts and, when necessary, rebels. It doesn't care about social trends, gender expectations or fashion. It operates on biological imperatives shaped over millennia and refined by evolution to thrive in conditions far removed from our modern world.

Today, we are witnessing subtle but undeniable shifts in human physiology, with women developing more body hair, men with declining sperm counts, rising infertility and widespread stress-related disorders.

These are important alarms.

Ban the F–Word

The phrase 'I'm fine' has affected more lives than every pandemic combined.

Patient Complaint: 'I'm fine'
Vitals: Denial elevated and self-awareness critically low
Diagnosis: Acute normalcy bias
Treatment Plan: Immediate truth serum

Varun's message read 'fine' when his vision narrowed while walking upstairs, telling himself it was just fatigue, low blood sugar or perhaps the consequence of a late night. He ignored the pounding in his chest, convincing himself it was nothing a strong coffee couldn't fix. However, that narrowing vision was his brain's way of signalling a need for oxygen, as blood vessels adjusted and pressure rose to help maintain balance. His body pleaded for attention, but his mind filed it under 'deal with later.'

Zara texted 'just tired' as her adrenal glands poured out cortisol, which is a stress hormone designed for life-or-death situations and not for stress related to overflowing email inboxes and performance reviews. Cortisol surged through her bloodstream, quickening her heartbeat, raising her blood pressure and gently tightening her blood vessels. Over time, chronic stress wore down her adrenal glands, challenged her immune system and strained her cardiovascular health. She dismissed it as burnout, too busy to acknowledge that her fight-or-flight response was never meant to be a 24/7 feature.

Abhishek laughed off his chest tightness, saying, 'It's probably indigestion. Perhaps I ate too quickly or something too spicy.' However, beneath his sternum, a serious situation was unfolding. The tightness in his chest indicated his heart's need for oxygen, as the coronary arteries narrowed or became partially blocked, with the risk of a clot or plaque disruption. Denial may have bought Abhishek some time to pursue other pressing matters, but not for his body.

Your body is a masterfully designed nuclear power station with 10,000 alarms working to keep you safe. Just tune in!

When Doing Everything Right Isn't Enough

The wellness industry has turned prevention into a moral imperative, creating an unspoken hierarchy where those who 'take responsibility' for their health are virtuous and those who fall ill are suspect. However, this mindset ignores fundamental truths.

Genetic Roulette: Your DNA carries hidden risks you can't fully control. That daily green smoothie won't change your BRCA genes and even perfect cholesterol levels don't guarantee completely clear arteries.

Environmental Wild Cards: You can't always control the air you breathe, the chemicals in your water or the viruses that quietly reside in your body. Pesticide drift from nearby farms, microplastics in your food and the long-term effects of everyday exposures happen regardless of your organic grocery choices.

Random Surprises: A single mutation in the wrong cell at the wrong time can shift the course of health. An unexpected infection can challenge multiple systems at once. Even a hidden vulnerability can surface suddenly, reminding us of the importance of vigilance and care.

When the Alarm Goes Unheard

The 2004 Indian Ocean tsunami, triggered by an undersea earthquake of 9.1-magnitude off the coast of Indonesia, struck the coastal areas of several countries in South Asia and Southeast Asia, giving rise to 100-foot waves. The tsunami's first sign, that is, the ocean's sudden retreat, went unheeded. Then came the impact. 230,000 lives were lost within minutes.[1]

Beep. Beep. Beeeeeep

The cardiac monitor's rhythmic pulse erupts into a single, piercing tone. A nurse slams the resuscitation trolley into place, her voice razor-sharp: 'He is arresting!'

On the hospital trolley, a 42-year-old finance director (who once emailed his doctor, 'Can we reschedule? The quarterly reports are due') now arches off the bed, with his ₹250,000 suit soaked in sweat. His pupils dilate as his left ventricle falters, starving itself of blood.

'Get the pads on him. NOW!'

Three hours earlier, he had laughed through lunch, rubbing his sternum: 'Must have overdone it at the gym.' Classic denial.

---

[1]Omer, Sevile, '2004 Indian Ocean Earthquake and Tsunami: Facts and FAQs', *World Vision*, 25 July 2025, https://tinyurl.com/mck86. Accessed on 8 December 2025.

What else did he miss?

- The 'acid reflux' that woke him at 3 a.m.
- The numbness in his left arm during presentations
- The exhaustion he blamed on 'burnout'

The defibrillator charges. His body convulses.

This is how modern ambition sometimes crumbles in open-plan offices, with Outlook notifications still pinging.

This Is Biological Mischief

Our ancestors evolved acute pain responses to survive predators and physical dangers. A surge of adrenaline heightened awareness and reflexes to ensure survival in the face of immediate danger.

However, we have become fluent in dismissing pain, mislabelling symptoms and rationalizing discomfort. We treat warning signs as glitches. We silence our body alarms by reclassifying them as 'nothing serious.'

Ironically, we have upgraded our phones fourteen times, each iteration more powerful than the last. Yet we run our bodies on 'Palaeolithic denialware,' which is a survival mechanism designed for quick, life-threatening scenarios, not for the persistent hum of chronic stress or unhealthy habits.

We silence physical alerts with pills, caffeine or self-reassurance. When a push notification arrives, we check it instantly, but a racing heart or chest pain? We swipe left.

From 'Hmm, That's Weird' to 'Okay, That's Important'

In an age obsessed with chasing an unattainable ideal of perfect health, we are going to do something radical in this book. We will learn how to understand and work with the bodies we actually have. Our bodies aren't trying to die, after all. Our bodies are trying to communicate. And knowing how to listen is just as important as knowing what to listen for.

In the coming chapters, we will take a head-to-toe approach—not as doctors diagnosing but as curious explorers mapping the body's signals.

By moving methodically from brain to heart, lungs to gut and muscles to skin, we will learn to decode their messages with clarity. Among other things, we will cover:

- When a headache is just a headache and when it's not
- Why skipped beats are usually harmless but persistent palpitations deserve attention
- The gut instincts
- The aches that mean 'rest' versus those that mean 'get this checked'

It's not about memorizing symptoms or self-diagnosing. It's about building a working relationship with your body where you know when to shrug off a twinge or when to take it seriously.

Let Us Understand Why We Respond the Way We Do

Human beings are remarkably adept at self-deception when it comes to health concerns. This tendency can seem irrational, but it is what it is.

The Normalcy Bias: 'It's Probably Nothing...'

Imagine you are experiencing a persistent headache or an unusual pain in your abdomen. Usually, your brain's first instinct is not to raise the alarm but to downplay it.

This reaction is called the normalcy bias. It is a cognitive distortion where the brain underestimates risks because acknowledging them feels overwhelming. It convinces you that unusual sensations are 'probably nothing' because admitting otherwise would push you to confront potential inconvenience.

This wiring often makes us dismiss:

- Chest tightness as 'gas'
- Recurrent headaches as 'excessive screen time'
- Unexplained weight loss as 'stress'

However, this response can sometimes delay action. During the 2004 Indian Ocean tsunami, many ignored the receding ocean, unaware that it was a warning sign. The normalcy bias can manifest similarly in health situations and keep people from addressing symptoms until later.

Nonetheless, understanding this bias can be quite empowering. Recognizing when your brain is minimizing a potential risk allows you to challenge it. Ask yourself: 'What if this isn't normal?' Developing this awareness can lead to early intervention and better outcomes.

The Productivity Paradox: 'I Can't Afford to Slow Down'

Across the world, working while unwell is often praised rather than questioned. Entrepreneurs, freelancers or homemakers often push through symptoms due to financial pressures, the fear of appearing weak or the belief that rest equates to laziness. Many parents and caregivers, too, ignore their own health to meet the needs of others.

The concept of 'powering through' is often glamourized. Statements like 'I don't have time to be sick' reflect a cultural mindset where ignoring symptoms is seen as resilience. This is the productivity paradox.

We applaud overwork while ignoring its costs. The consequence? A decline in performance, increased stress and sometimes greater health challenges.

Globally, presenteeism, or working while sick, costs economies billions in lost productivity.[2]

The Familiarity Trap: 'I Know My Body'

Humans thrive on routine. The predictability of daily life offers a sense of control and comfort. Disrupting that by acknowledging a potential health issue feels like inviting trouble. This tendency is especially strong in people juggling multiple roles who already feel overwhelmed. Taking a break to address a health concern feels like letting a fragile balance slip.

A study in *Psychosomatic Medicine* found that individuals with high stress levels often interpret physical symptoms as stress-related rather than medical, thereby delaying proper care.[3]

The Social Comparison Trap: 'They Are Coping, So Should I'

Social comparison is a fundamental human behaviour. We constantly gauge our own efforts against colleagues working late, friends juggling responsibilities, influencers flaunting productivity, and others. This creates a distorted benchmark.

---

[2]Evans-Lacko, Sara, and Martin Knapp, 'Global Patterns of Workplace Productivity for People with Depression: Absenteeism and Presenteeism Costs across Eight Diverse Countries', *Social Psychiatry and Psychiatric Epidemiology*, Vol. 51, No. 11, 2016, pp. 1525–37, https://doi.org/10.1007/s00127-016-1278-4. Accessed on 8 December 2025.

[3]Cameron, Linda, Elaine A. Leventhal, and Howard Leventhal, 'Seeking Medical Care in Response to Symptoms and Life Stress', *Psychosomatic Medicine*, Vol. 57, No. 1, 1995, pp. 37–47, https://doi.org/10.1097/00006842-199501000-00006. Accessed on 8 December 2025.

Seeing others seemingly handle pressure without faltering can make us question our own resilience.

However, what is often unseen are the breakdowns, burnout episodes and silent health struggles behind the scenes. Comparing your personal limits to others' is misleading. Everyone has unique thresholds and pushing beyond yours simply to 'keep up' is a recipe for harm in some cases.

The Optimism Bias: 'It Won't Happen to Me'

Psychologically, many believe that severe health issues happen to 'other' people. This phenomenon, called the optimism bias, often leads to underestimating personal risk. People assume that because they have been fine so far, they will continue to be.

This sense of invincibility is especially prevalent among young people. Many young professionals enter high-pressure jobs early, sacrificing sleep, skipping meals and working relentless hours. The absence of major health issues so far convinces them that they are naturally resilient.

However, studies show that chronic sleep deprivation alone can increase the risk of cardiovascular problems by 45 per cent.[4]

The Manifestation Myth: 'If I Ignore It, It Won't Happen'

The belief in 'speaking things into existence' has inspired

---

[4]Cappuccio, Francesco P., Daniel Cooper, Lanfranco D'Elia, Pasquale Strazzullo, and Michelle A. Miller, 'Sleep Duration Predicts Cardiovascular Outcomes: A Systematic Review and Meta-Analysis of Prospective Studies', *European Heart Journal*, Vol. 32, No. 12, 2011, pp. 1484–94, https://doi.org/10.1093/eurheartj/ehr007; Liberman, Joshua, 'Prioritizing Health | Sleep and Cardiovascular Health', *American College of Cardiology*, 1 March 2025, https://tinyurl.com/5fccekep. Accessed on 10 December 2025.

many to harness the power of positive thinking. However, this mindset can also backfire when taken to extremes, particularly when it comes to health. Some people avoid acknowledging symptoms, fearing that simply naming an illness will somehow manifest it into reality.

Phrases like:

- 'I won't claim this sickness.'
- 'I'm not sick, it's just stress.'
- 'If I don't think about it, it will go away.'

...can become dangerous forms of denial. While optimism is valuable, ignoring symptoms doesn't prevent illness but instead delays treatment.

The Sexual Stigma: 'It's Too Embarrassing to Discuss'

Sexual health remains one of the most shrouded in silence, not because it is unimportant but because it is steeped in shame, cultural taboos and deep-seated discomfort. From erectile dysfunction to unexplained pelvic pain, people routinely ignore or downplay symptoms, fearing judgement from doctors, partners and even themselves.

The result? Treatable conditions sometimes escalate into chronic pain, infertility or even life-threatening illnesses, all because embarrassment was louder than the body's alarms.

The Insurance Illusion: 'It's Just a Bill I Can't Pay Right Now'

For millions around the world, healthcare is a financial tightrope walk as much as it is a matter of access. In countries where medical care is prohibitively expensive or insurance coverage is unreliable, people often tend to ignore symptoms, hoping that the symptoms will simply go away.

A cough? Probably nothing. A lingering fever? Wait it

out. The fear isn't just illness itself. It's the bills that follow.

Further, when healthcare is a luxury and the system feels rigged, people stop seeing doctors as allies and start seeing them as financial predators. Thus, what starts as a manageable issue can sometimes spiral into a full-blown crisis by the time they finally seek help.

The Sunk Cost Fallacy: 'I Have Already Invested Too Much to Stop Now'

Humans are wired to hate losing more than they love winning, and nowhere is this more counterproductive than when it comes to their health, time and well-being. The sunk cost fallacy tricks us into clinging to failing endeavours, toxic habits and unsustainable lifestyles, simply because we have already 'invested' too much to walk away.

- 'I have worked 80-hour weeks for years. If I slow down now, it was all for nothing.'
- 'I have handled everything alone this long. Asking for help means that I have failed.'
- 'If I take a break now, it will mean that I am abandoning them.'

Every moment spent clinging to a sinking ship is a moment you could have spent swimming to shore.

Real strength is defined less by endurance and more by the courage to sometimes let go.

The Faith Fallacy: 'God Will Heal Me'

In many deeply religious communities, there exists an assumption that seeking medical treatment demonstrates a lack of faith and that true believers should rely solely on prayer for healing. While faith can provide profound emotional strength and even contribute to recovery, it becomes a perilous trap when used as a substitute for medical intervention.[5]

To ignore medical help when it is available is, instead of piety, a gamble with the very life faith seeks to preserve.

- A diabetic refuses insulin, a cancer patient delays chemo, or a heart attack victim rejects the ER (all in the name of faith).
- Religious exemptions allow preventable tragedies from measles, meningitis and untreated infections.
- Depression, schizophrenia and anxiety disorders go untreated and are labelled as 'demonic' spiritual failings rather than medical conditions.

The Google Effect: 'I Can Figure This Out Myself!'

The Google effect, that is, the tendency to rely on search engines instead of professional advice, often leads people down a rabbit hole of misinformation.

We have all been there:

- Search 'night sweat causes'
- Jump from 'menopause' to 'TB' to 'lymphoma' in 0.4 seconds
- Land on 'Maybe it's vitamin D deficiency?'
- Order supplements instead of seeing a doctor

The internet is a powerful tool, but when it comes to health, it might not be that powerful.

---

[5]University of Rochester Medical Centre, 'Cancer and Spirituality', *URMC Health Encyclopaedia*, https://tinyurl.com/mv2ew2j9. Accessed on 11 September 2025.

The Art of Body Literacy

It is a dangerous illusion that we can control or micromanage every aspect of our health, emotions or bodily functions. However, if control is an illusion, where does that leave us? Should we swing to the opposite extreme—ignoring signals, dismissing discomfort and resigning ourselves to fate?

The answer lies in cultivating body literacy. It's the ability to listen to your body's signals without spiralling into anxiety. It's about being alert but not anxious. It's a skill that requires both knowledge and emotional balance.

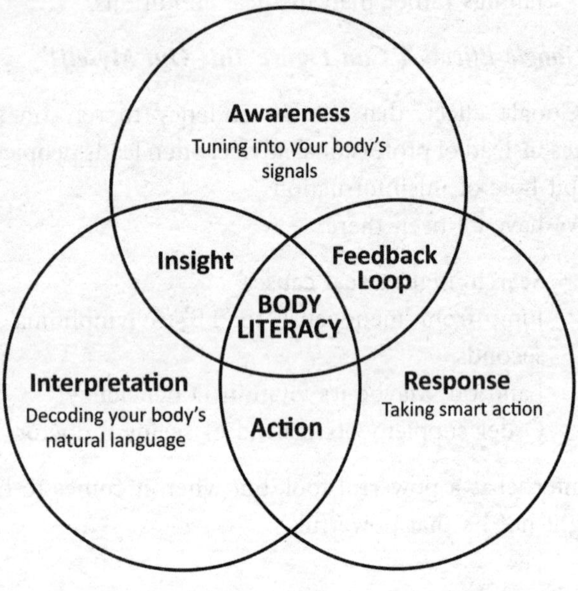

Figure 1: The three pillars of body literacy

Three Pillars of Body Literacy

Awareness: Tuning Into Your Body's Signals

Most of us operate on autopilot and ignore subtle cues until they escalate. Awareness is the practice of checking in with our body before something feels 'off.'

- **Daily Body Scans:** Take five minutes to mentally scan from head to toe. Notice tension, discomfort or energy shifts.
- **Recognize Your Baseline:** What's normal for you? (For example, some people naturally have cold hands, while others have warm hands.)
- **Track Patterns, Not Just Symptoms:** Does your back always hurt after sitting too long? Does caffeine make your heart race?

Interpretation: Decoding Your Body's Natural Language

A sensation is just a signal. It doesn't always mean potential risk. Interpretation is the skill of distinguishing between:

- Normal fluctuations (for example, temporary fatigue from poor sleep)
- Benign quirks (for example, harmless muscle twitches)
- Legitimate red flags (for example, sudden, unexplained weight loss)

If a symptom happens three times in a short span or lasts three days, investigate.

Did the dizziness start after a new medication? Did the rash appear after eating something new?

Response: Taking Smart Action

Once you detect and interpret a signal, the next step is response, that is, knowing when to:

- Wait and observe (most minor issues resolve on their own)
- Adjust lifestyle (for example, more water, better sleep and stress management)
- Seek professional input (in case the symptoms are persistent, severe or escalating)

Keep a symptom log. Note timing, triggers and severity. Doctors find this far more useful than vague descriptions.

PART 2

RECOGNIZING SPECIFIC BODY ALARMS

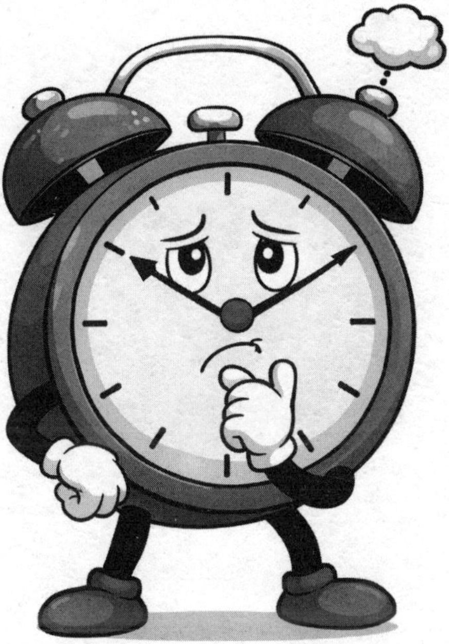

When Your Head's Got Its Act Together

A healthy head feels comfortable and responsive without unusual tension or discomfort. The scalp is smooth and free from tenderness, bumps and flaky patches and the hair feels full and evenly dense. Your face moves symmetrically with natural expressions and your skin is clear, without sudden spots and unusual changes.

The eyes are bright, pupils react evenly to light, and the whites remain clear and free of yellowing. Ears feel clear and unblocked. Your jaw opens and closes smoothly and your gums are firm and pink. The tongue rests relaxed and moist, with a healthy colour and texture. Breathing flows deeply and effortlessly through the nose and mouth. Mentally, the mind feels clear, calm and focused, reflecting a balanced connection between body and brain.

This is the head's natural state. Alert, comfortable and quietly protecting you every moment. If it doesn't feel this way, your head could be sounding the first alarm. Tune in.

Health Has a Face, and It's Yours

The human head is a relentless whistleblower, revealing secrets the body would rather keep hidden. Every twitch, every discolouration and every asymmetry is a coded message, leading to truths that could make a difference.

Consider the scalp. Most regard it as nothing more than a foundation for hair. However, its texture, its lesions and its very topography can reflect conditions long before blood tests catch up. A shifting hairline may be influenced by genetics, yes, but it can also be shaped by hormones or thyroid activity. A persistent itch could be dandruff or it could be the body's way of nudging us to investigate further. The evidence is there, visible and tangible, if one knows where to look.

The face is also a ledger of hidden truths. Forehead creases are not just the etchings of time, they can also map chronic dehydration or even cardiovascular strain. A drooping eyelid may be nothing, or it may be the earliest signal of a neurological or muscular condition. The eyes, often called windows to the soul, are equally windows to the liver, the kidneys and even the brain.

Then, there is the mouth. Bleeding gums may simply reflect brushing too hard or they may be signalling nutritional gaps or systemic concerns. Persistent sores deserve a second look. The jaw clicks and the teeth grind are signs of stress but also of sleep apnoea, which is linked to heart disease.

This chapter invites readers to look again at what they see in the mirror each morning. Often, the first signs of imbalance are not visible in lab results, but in the simple act of paying attention.

Making Peace with the Headache

Headaches are a universal experience that nearly everyone has encountered at some point. However, not all headaches are created equal. While most are benign, others can be a sign of something much more serious. Understanding the nature of your headache, its accompanying symptoms and its patterns is crucial for distinguishing between a common tension headache and a potentially life-threatening condition.

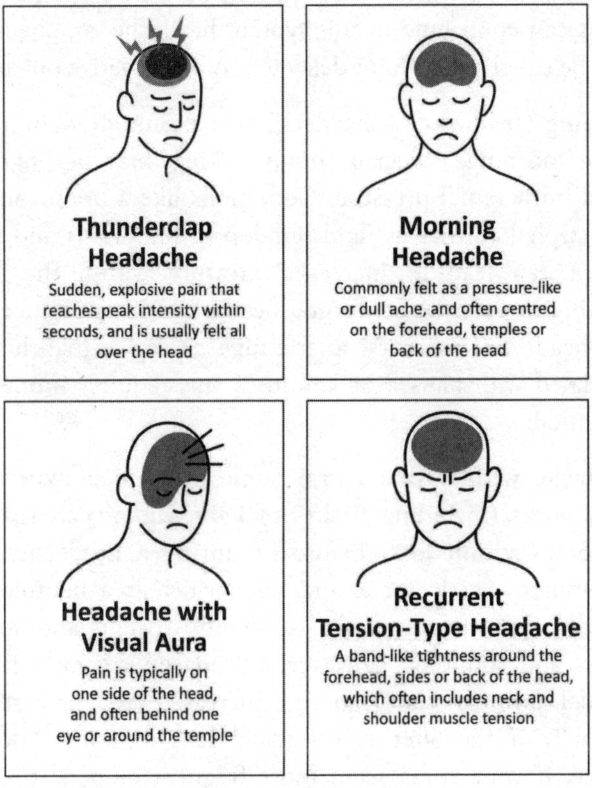

Figure 2: Types of headaches

Types of Headaches and Their Implications

Thunderclap Headache: Often described as the worst headache of your life, a thunderclap headache comes on suddenly, without warning and peaks within minutes. This severe, intense pain can be a sign of an aneurysm (that is, a bulging blood vessel in the brain) and should be treated as a medical emergency until proven otherwise. While other causes can contribute to this type of headache, an aneurysm must be ruled out without delay to prevent negative outcomes.

Morning Headache: A headache that occurs predominantly in the morning, especially upon waking, may be linked to raised intracranial pressure. Conditions like a brain tumour, hydrocephalus (that is, fluid buildup in the brain) and sleep apnoea can lead to increased pressure within the skull, resulting in persistent morning headaches. If you notice that your headaches are worse after a night's sleep or that they are associated with nausea or vomiting, this requires immediate evaluation.

Headache with Visual Aura: Some individuals experience visual auras (including flashes of light, zigzag patterns and temporary vision loss) before or during a headache. This symptom is classic for a migraine, which is a neurological disorder that often involves sensitivity to light and sound, nausea and vomiting. However, a headache accompanied by a visual aura can also signal an increased risk for a stroke, especially if the aura is unusually long-lasting or doesn't resolve. If your auras seem more frequent or persist longer than normal, it is important to consult a doctor.

Recurrent Tension-Type Headaches: These are the most common forms of headache, often caused by stress, poor posture and muscle tension. These headaches tend to be less severe but more persistent, often affecting the forehead, temples and neck. They may be linked to environmental factors, such as long hours at a desk, staring at a screen and even a lack of sleep. Chronic tension-type headaches may also indicate an underlying problem with lifestyle or mental health, such as anxiety and depression. Adopting better ergonomic practices, managing stress and improving sleep hygiene can often alleviate these headaches.

When Headaches Are More Than Just a Headache

Headache with Fever and Stiff Neck: This combination of symptoms is classic for meningitis, which is an infection of the protective membranes surrounding the brain and spinal cord. Meningitis can cause severe, rapidly progressing symptoms and may require urgent medical attention. Early diagnosis and treatment are essential for the best outcomes.

Headache with Sudden Neurological Symptoms: If a headache is accompanied by sudden changes in mental status, motor function and vision, this could indicate a stroke, seizure or a serious brain condition. Prompt medical evaluation is crucial for accurate diagnosis and timely care.

There Is More to Headaches Than Meets the Nerve

Understanding headaches is not just about identifying the pain. It is also about recognizing the context in which the pain occurs. For example, chronic tension-type headaches often indicate a lifestyle imbalance and migraines may signal an underlying neurovascular disorder. Further, the sudden onset of an intense headache, particularly if it differs from your usual patterns, could indicate something far more serious, such as an aneurysm or stroke.

People with a history of migraine may experience different types of migraine episodes over time. Migraines can evolve in severity and frequency and understanding these shifts can help doctors provide better treatments. Additionally, modern imaging technology has vastly improved our ability to diagnose conditions like raised intracranial pressure, strokes and aneurysms, making timely diagnosis and intervention possible.

Therefore, listen carefully to your body, and if something doesn't feel right, don't hesitate to seek professional guidance.

Reading the Scalp's Language

When you think of your scalp, you probably just think of hair. But your scalp is much more than that. It is a living and breathing part of your body that can reveal early signs of deeper health issues. Itching, flaking, sudden hair loss or irritation can actually be your body's quiet way of saying, 'Pay attention. Something is not right.'

Dandruff or Something More?

Most people have dealt with annoying white flakes on their shirt collar and the occasional itch at some point. It is usually caused by a natural yeast that lives on our skin and while it can be embarrassing, it is not dangerous.

Having said that, when the flakes get greasy or yellow, or the itching becomes more intense and spreads beyond your scalp to your eyebrows, sides of the nose and even your chest, you might be dealing with seborrhoeic dermatitis. It is like dandruff's bigger, messier cousin. And unlike regular dandruff, it involves inflammation. Your skin is actually reacting and getting irritated, and it is not just shedding.

Dandruff	*Seborrhoeic Dermatitis*
Dry, white flakes	Oily, yellowish flakes
Mild itching	More intense itching and redness
Only on the scalp	Can spread to the face, chest and ears

If the condition keeps coming back, especially if you have a medical condition like Parkinson's disease or a weakened immune system, it is worth checking in with a doctor.

Scalp Psoriasis: When It's More Than Skin Deep

Sometimes, what looks like 'just a flaky scalp' is actually something more serious. Psoriasis. This is a condition where the immune system causes the skin to grow too fast, leading to thick, scaly patches. These patches can itch, hurt and sometimes even bleed when scratched.

Psoriasis on the scalp can be one of the first signs of the condition, even before you notice any other symptoms on your body. And it is not just a skin issue. Psoriasis is linked to other health risks as well, like joint pain, heart problems and even depression.

What to watch for:

- Thick, silver-coloured scales that feel different from regular dandruff
- Well-defined patches that don't go away easily
- Small areas of bleeding if you pick or scratch
- Family history of psoriasis or autoimmune diseases

If this sounds familiar, early diagnosis and intervention can help manage symptoms and prevent complications.

Sudden Hair Loss?

Waking up to find a round, bald patch on your scalp can be concerning, but it doesn't always mean something serious. One possible cause is alopecia areata, which is a condition where the immune system mistakenly targets hair follicles. It often appears suddenly and may result in small, smooth, hairless patches on the scalp or other parts of the body. While it can occasionally lead to more widespread hair loss, many cases are temporary, manageable and even reversible with care and support.

When an Itchy Scalp Has More to Say

Everyone experiences an itchy scalp from time to time. Most of the time, it's nothing to worry about and settles on its own. However, if the itching continues despite changes in haircare or comes with other noticeable changes, it may be your body's way of nudging you to pay closer attention.

Some possible underlying causes include:

- Fungal infections, especially in children, which may show as broken hairs or tiny black dots
- Allergic reactions to hair dyes, styling products or harsh shampoos
- Thyroid disorders, which can lead to dry, brittle hair or excessive shedding
- Iron or zinc deficiency, which may impact hair and skin health
- Liver or kidney issues, which sometimes cause generalized itchiness

If the discomfort lingers for more than a couple of weeks or comes with other changes in your body, a simple check-up and basic blood work can help rule things out and offer peace of mind.

When to Check in with a Doctor

- **Still struggling after two to three weeks of treatment?** It's best not to keep switching shampoos. Instead, consider consulting a healthcare professional who can help you get to the root of the issue.
- **Oozing, crusting or sore spots on your scalp?** These could signal an infection or, in some cases, an underlying skin condition that deserves a closer look.
- **Tiredness, weight loss or joint pain alongside scalp issues?** These symptoms might point to a thyroid imbalance or an autoimmune condition such as lupus. A simple check-up can provide clarity.

The Forehead Story

Your forehead does more than just wrinkle with emotion. It quietly tells stories about your health, habits and sometimes even hidden illnesses. Whether it's a deep furrow, a recurring spot or a changing mole, the forehead is often one of the first places where internal imbalances make a visible appearance.

What Your Forehead Lines Reveal

We all get forehead lines as we age, especially from repeated facial expressions, sun exposure and thinning skin. Some say that each line tells a story of worry, wisdom or years of squinting into the sun without sunscreen. In certain cultures, deep forehead lines are even seen as signs of intelligence and good fortune.

Still, science offers a slightly less romantic take. Prominent horizontal forehead lines, particularly in younger individuals, have been linked to chronic stress and elevated cortisol levels. More intriguingly, a 2018 French study published in the *European Journal of Cardiology* observed that deep forehead wrinkles might correlate with an increased risk of cardiovascular disease, possibly due to microvascular changes in the skin.[6]

So, while they may earn you points in a palm reader's booth or a few approving nods from elders, they are worth paying attention to, especially if you also have other cardiovascular risk factors like hypertension, diabetes or a strong family history of these diseases.

Not All Moles Are Harmless

Forehead moles are common, but when they change in colour, shape or texture, they demand attention. The ABCDE rule is a helpful way to assess whether a mole or skin lesion may be suspicious.

Letter	*What It Stands For*	*What to Watch For*
A	Asymmetry	One half unlike the other
B	Border	Irregular, blurred or notched edges
C	Colour	Multiple shades or sudden darkening

[6]Esquirol, Y., J. Ferrieres, J.C. Marquie, S. Huo Yung Kai, M. Niezborala, E. Berard, V. Bongard, J.B. Ruidavets, and the VISAT group, 'Forehead Wrinkles and Risk of All-Cause and Cardiovascular Mortality over 20-Year Follow-Up in a Working Population: VISAT Study', *European Heart Journal*, Vol. 39, Suppl. 1, 2018, p. 1548, https://doi.org/10.1093/eurheartj/ehy565.P1548. Accessed on 8 December 2025.

Letter	*What It Stands For*	*What to Watch For*
D	Diameter	Larger than 6 mm (about the size of a pencil eraser)
E	Evolving	Any change in size, shape, colour or symptoms

Moles that itch, bleed, crust over or appear suddenly should be examined by a dermatologist. While such changes can be harmless, they can also be early signs of melanoma, which is the most serious type of skin cancer. The good news is that when caught early, melanoma is highly treatable and outcomes are often excellent.

More Than Meets the Eye

We blink them open each morning without a second thought. We blame screens for their tiredness, rub them when stressed and ignore subtle changes until the world looks different through them. The human eye is a delicate, complex structure—constantly exposed to the elements—and is tightly interwoven with multiple systems in the body. Often, it is one of the first places where subtle internal imbalances begin to surface.

Yellowing of the Whites

The whites of your eyes, known as the sclerae, are naturally meant to remain, well, white. However, when they take on a yellowish hue, it is not just a sign of a few sleepless nights or a bit of fatigue. This subtle change may serve as your body's early warning system, pointing to deeper concerns worth checking.

Here are a few potential causes behind yellowing sclerae:

Liver Disorders: Conditions like hepatitis and cirrhosis can impair the liver and stop it from filtering waste properly. This leads to a buildup of bilirubin (a yellow substance), which can make the whites of your eyes look yellow.

Bile Duct Blockage: Blockages in the bile ducts, sometimes caused by gallstones, can interfere with the normal flow of bile, triggering that yellowish tint in the eyes, long before the skin shows noticeable signs of jaundice.

Excessive Breakdown of Red Blood Cells (Haemolysis): When red blood cells break down too quickly due to certain conditions or disorders, excess bilirubin builds up in the blood. This can cause yellowing of the eyes and skin as the body struggles to remove the waste.

If the whites of your eyes begin to look yellow, it is not necessarily a cause for alarm, but it is reason enough to check in with a healthcare professional.

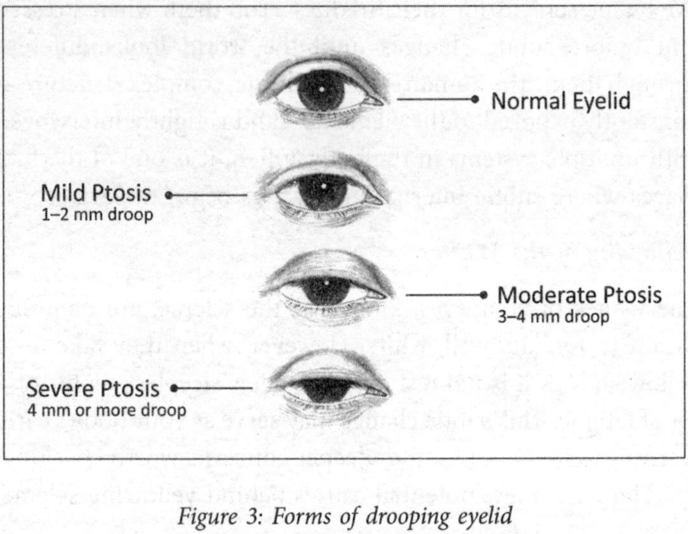

Figure 3: Forms of drooping eyelid

Drooping Eyelid

A sagging upper eyelid, known as ptosis, may seem like just a sign of ageing or fatigue, but when it develops suddenly or unevenly, it could indicate a more serious underlying condition. If you notice one or both eyelids drooping, it is important to pay attention. Here are some potential causes:

Myasthenia Gravis: This autoimmune disorder affects the communication between the nerves and muscles, leading to weakness in voluntary muscles. Ptosis is a common symptom of this condition and may occur alongside other signs like double vision and difficulty swallowing.

Nerve Compression: Conditions like Horner's syndrome can cause ptosis due to damage to the sympathetic nerves that control the muscles around the eye. This can also result in other symptoms such as pupil constriction and reduced sweating on one side of the face.

Transient Ischaemic Attack (Mini-Stroke): Sudden ptosis, especially when combined with other symptoms like slurred speech, weakness in the face or limbs and difficulty speaking, may point to a mini-stroke. A TIA can cause temporary disruptions in blood flow to the brain, which can impact muscle control, including the muscles around your eyes.

If you experience ptosis along with other neurological signs, such as weakness on one side of the face or body and changes in vision, seek medical attention without delay. These could be signs of a serious underlying condition, and early evaluation can make a meaningful difference.

That Little Eyelid Twitch?

We have all experienced that pesky eyelid twitch, usually

blamed on stress, lack of sleep or an extra shot of espresso. And in most cases, we are right. However, when the twitching lingers, worsens or spreads beyond the eye, it might signal something more.

A magnesium deficiency, for instance, can lead to involuntary muscle spasms, including eye twitching, as this mineral is key to muscle control. Chronic stress can also overload your nervous system, causing frequent or intense twitches. In rarer cases, persistent twitching that affects other facial muscles may point to neurological irritation or a movement disorder.

Ensure that you are getting enough magnesium, especially if you are prone to muscle spasms. Foods like leafy greens, nuts, seeds and whole grains are excellent sources. If chronic stress is the culprit, explore relaxation techniques such as yoga, meditation and deep breathing exercises.

When the World Blurs, Listen to Your Eyes

Any sudden changes in your vision, whether it is blurriness, double vision or difficulty focusing, deserve attention. These early shifts may be your body's way of signalling underlying health concerns, including:

Diabetic Retinopathy: This is one of the leading causes of vision loss and is closely linked to poorly controlled blood sugar levels. Over time, high blood sugar can damage the blood vessels in the retina, causing vision issues. Early detection and proper diabetes management can significantly reduce the risk.

Glaucoma: Often referred to as the 'silent thief of sight,' glaucoma involves damage to the optic nerve, usually due to increased pressure within the eye. What makes it especially tricky is that it can progress without obvious symptoms at first. Early warning signs, such as blurred vision or seeing halos around lights, should never be overlooked.

Retinal Detachment: This occurs when the retina (which is the light-sensitive tissue at the back of the eye) becomes separated from its supporting tissues. Symptoms often start with flashes of light, the sudden appearance of floaters and a curtain-like shadow in your peripheral vision. Though it sounds alarming, prompt medical treatment can often restore vision or prevent long-term damage. So, don't delay going to the doctor.

Stroke: A stroke can affect your vision, causing partial or complete loss of vision on one side of your field of vision. In some cases, vision loss may occur suddenly, along with other neurological symptoms like facial weakness and slurred speech.

Your vision is precious, and even subtle changes shouldn't be overlooked. Always take action if you notice anything unusual with your vision. Clarity should never be compromised.

Redness, Pain and Light Sensitivity

A red eye might seem like a common and minor issue, but the context is crucial. Is it merely itchy and watery, like with seasonal allergies? Or is it accompanied by pain, light sensitivity and blurry vision? Understanding the difference can be vital in diagnosing the problem and preventing any complications.

Conjunctivitis: Often caused by either an infection (bacterial or viral) or an allergy, conjunctivitis results in redness, irritation and discharge. While it is usually not serious, it can spread easily and cause discomfort, especially if left untreated.

Uveitis: This condition involves inflammation of the uvea, which is the middle layer of the eye. It is often associated with autoimmune diseases and can lead to severe pain, light sensitivity and blurred vision. With timely medical care, most people recover well and avoid lasting damage.

Keratitis: This refers to inflammation of the cornea, often due to infection. It is particularly common in contact lens wearers, especially if lenses are not cleaned properly or are worn for extended periods. While keratitis can be painful and serious, early diagnosis and treatment usually lead to full recovery and help preserve clear vision.

Over-the-counter eye drops may offer temporary relief but using them without a proper diagnosis can delay necessary treatment and may worsen the condition. Don't rely on them if you are experiencing pain or other severe symptoms. Always err on the side of caution when your eyes are in distress.

What Lies behind Dark Circles

Dark circles beneath the eyes are more than a sign of a late night. While they often result from fatigue, genetics and dehydration, persistent under-eye darkness may also hint at poor circulation, nutritional deficiencies or even chronic allergies.

These shadows occur when the delicate skin under the eyes thins over time, allowing the underlying blood vessels to show through. This phenomenon, though common, may be exacerbated by factors such as stress, lack of sleep and a diet low in essential vitamins and iron. In some cases, the presence of dark circles suggests that lifestyle adjustments or further medical evaluation might be necessary.

Your Nose Knows Best

We breathe in silence thousands of times each day, seldom noticing the gateway that makes it possible: the nose. Tucked neatly at the centre of our face, this seemingly simple organ does far more than just sniff aromas or wrinkle in disdain. It is the first line of defence against airborne invaders and a sensitive alarm system (if we listen closely). A little congestion here, an occasional bleed there, a lost scent or a stuffy child's voice—these symptoms may be brushed aside as minor nuisances, but at times they are far more telling.

The Invisible Burden of Chronic Congestion

Chronic nasal stuffiness is one of the most underappreciated disruptions to quality of life. Many live with it for years, assuming it is normal. However, prolonged congestion is the body raising a quiet hand for attention. Two common causes emerge:

Allergies: Often seasonal but increasingly perennial, allergic rhinitis is an immune overreaction to harmless substances like pollen, dust mites and animal dander. It brings with it sneezing fits, itchy eyes and a runny or blocked nose.

Nasal Polyps: These soft, painless, noncancerous growths arise from chronic inflammation. They narrow or block the nasal passages and are often mistaken for allergies. When congestion persists despite antihistamines, polyps deserve suspicion. Polyps are more likely if:

- You breathe better on one side of your nose
- You snore or mouth-breathe at night
- You have asthma or aspirin sensitivity (a part of the 'Samter's Triad')

The body does not block its own airways without reason. Chronic congestion, especially when resistant to standard treatment, is never something to 'just live with.' Find the reason, and the relief will follow.

When the Nose Bleeds, Listen Closely

Nosebleeds, or epistaxis, are common, especially in dry climates and during seasonal changes. However, frequent or severe nosebleeds are not always innocent. Two hidden causes demand close attention:

High Blood Pressure: Hypertension can make blood vessels in the nose fragile and prone to rupture. In older adults, a sudden nosebleed may be the first visible sign of elevated blood pressure.

Bleeding Disorders: In children or young adults, frequent bleeds may be an early symptom of a clotting abnormality. Conditions like Von Willebrand disease (VWD) or platelet dysfunctions may lurk behind what seems like 'just another nosebleed.'

Be alert when:

- Bleeding occurs without trauma
- It lasts longer than 10 minutes
- It is associated with bruising elsewhere on the body

If nosebleeds are frequent, unexplained or difficult to stop, it is important to get them medically evaluated for clarity.

When Smell Disappears, So Does Warning

Loss of smell, or anosmia, gained global attention during the COVID-19 pandemic. However, while viruses are a leading cause, and often reversible, persistent smell loss can signal deeper issues:

- COVID-19 (often sudden, usually reversible)
- Parkinson's disease (anosmia may precede motor symptoms by years)
- Zinc deficiency (a silent nutritional shortfall with widespread consequences on taste, immunity and healing)

Persistent smell loss is not only about missing perfumes or food aromas. It endangers your safety. For example, you might not smell a gas leak, smoke in the case of fire, or spoiled food. It may also hint at neurodegeneration or metabolic imbalances. If the smell doesn't return within a few weeks after a viral illness, consult a healthcare provider.

When a Child Speaks through Their Nose

A child with a nasal voice, frequent mouth breathing or snoring might be more than just 'a bit congested.' These signs can point to enlarged adenoids, tonsils and structural issues (like a deviated nasal septum). Over time, chronic mouth breathing in children can alter facial development, affect speech and impair sleep and concentration.

All this is more than ENT (ear, nose and throat) territory. It is a developmental issue. Children who breathe through their mouths are often misdiagnosed with attention issues or poor behaviour when, in fact, they are simply oxygen deprived.

Don't ignore:

- Daytime fatigue despite full sleep
- Breathing pauses during sleep
- A flat or long face with a narrow jaw (signs of chronic oral breathing)

In such cases, an ENT evaluation can be life-changing.

The Ear Deserves to Be Heard Too

Ever had that strange ringing in your ears after a loud concert? Or felt like the room was spinning for no reason? Maybe you have woken up with a blocked ear, as if an invisible hand pressed the mute button on the world. These are your ears sending you urgent messages. Think of your ears as your body's built-in surveillance system. They don't just hear. They listen to your blood pressure, to your stress levels and even to the pressure inside your skull.

The Ringing You Shouldn't Ignore

A soft ringing, a high-pitched buzz, a faint hiss…when sounds appear without an external source, your ears are trying to tell you something. This phenomenon, known as tinnitus, is often shrugged off as harmless, but it can be the body's early alert system. Sometimes, it is a sign of hearing loss creeping in, brought on by age or repeated exposure to loud environments. Other times, it reflects deeper issues, such as stress, poor circulation and conditions like Ménière's disease affecting the inner ear. If the noise arrives suddenly or begins to grow louder, don't tune it out. Early awareness opens doors to relief.

Ear Pain while Chewing or Speaking

If your ear aches every time you chew, yawn or even speak, it might not be the ear itself that is to blame. The real issue could lie in the temporomandibular joint (TMJ), which is the complex hinge that connects your jaw to your skull. TMJ dysfunction can trigger referred pain that radiates into the ear, mimicking an ear infection or blockage.

Similarly, dental problems like abscesses, impacted wisdom teeth and bruxism (that is, teeth grinding) can create a ripple effect, resulting in pain perceived as coming from the ear. These overlapping pain pathways show just how interconnected your head and neck anatomy really is. Sometimes, treating an earache means starting with the dentist or jaw specialist, rather than the audiologist.

Unexpected Ear Discharge

While ear discharge isn't uncommon, especially in young children with middle ear infections, it should never be casually dismissed. The key lies in observing what kind of fluid is leaking, when it occurs and what else is happening alongside it.

One of the most frequent causes is otitis media, which is a middle ear infection that can lead to a buildup of fluid behind the eardrum. When the pressure becomes too intense, the eardrum may rupture, releasing a pus-like fluid. Interestingly, this may even bring momentary relief from pain, but it still warrants prompt medical review and follow-up care.

Furthermore, not all discharges are created equal. A thin, clear and watery fluid, especially if it appears after head trauma or a recent surgery, could signal a cerebrospinal fluid (CSF) leak (a rare but serious condition where the protective barrier around the brain is compromised).

Even a small amount of blood-tinged fluid, particularly without visible injury, is worth investigating. The ear has its own way of asking for care, and with timely evaluation, most causes can be resolved safely and effectively.

Dizziness and Disorientation

The inner ear does more than just catch sound. It also acts as your body's silent stabilizer, guiding your sense of balance and spatial awareness. Nestled within this intricate structure is the vestibular system, which is a delicate but powerful internal compass. When it falters, the world can feel like it is shifting beneath your feet, sometimes literally.

Occasional light-headedness or brief dizziness can be harmless as it is often linked to fatigue, dehydration, low blood pressure and standing up too quickly. However, when these sensations become sudden, recurrent or intense, they could signal an underlying issue in the inner ear.

If you ever feel as though the room is spinning or your steps are uncertain, it may not be inside your head but inside your ear. Don't dismiss it as clumsiness or a rough day. Your internal gyroscope might be struggling to keep up.

Importantly, balance-related symptoms are sometimes misattributed to anxiety or general stress, especially in younger adults. While stress can exacerbate dizziness, it is worth investigating whether the root cause lies deeper within the labyrinth of the inner ear.

The Non-Negotiables

- Sudden hearing loss, especially in one ear, is a medical emergency. When treated within 24 to 72 hours, there is often a good chance of restoring hearing and preventing long-term damage.
- Unexplained discharge, particularly clear or blood-tinged fluid, should be investigated without delay.
- Vertigo accompanied by vomiting, double vision and facial weakness may indicate a neurological emergency. While it may sometimes be linked to inner ear disturbances as well, such combinations of symptoms should be evaluated promptly.

SOS from the Mouth

Often overlooked in clinical assessments, the mouth is, in fact, a microcosm of internal health. Its structures—including the tongue, gums, mucosa, lips and salivary glands—are sensitive to the body's nutritional state, hormonal shifts, inflammatory markers and even neurological integrity. Every ulcer that lingers, every coating that thickens and every change in breath or taste has a tale to tell.

While a skin rash or a fever often triggers immediate concern, oral symptoms are more likely to be dismissed and brushed aside as trivial or temporary. However, conditions such as iron-deficiency anaemia, vitamin B12 depletion, type 2 diabetes, renal or hepatic dysfunction and even early malignancies can quietly surface through subtle changes in the mouth.

Moreover, the oral cavity is deeply interconnected with the gastrointestinal tract and the immune system. From the tongue's texture to the breath's odour and from gum integrity to mucosal tone, each detail contributes to a larger physiological portrait if we know how to read it.

The Tongue Talks

The next time you look in the mirror, take a closer look at your tongue. Check your tongue in natural light, ideally in the morning before brushing, for a more accurate snapshot of your internal state. The tongue is a bio-indicator, revealing information about hydration status, immunity, nutrient levels and microbial health. When interpreted correctly, it can serve as an early diagnostic tool.

Tongue Sign	*What It May Indicate*	*Why You Shouldn't Ignore It*
Thick white coating	Fungal overgrowth or microbial imbalance	Restoring oral and gut health now can prevent deeper infections
Smooth or beefy-red appearance	Nutritional deficiency affecting mucosal regeneration	Spotting this can help correct deficiencies early, before fatigue or nerve issues begin
Cracks at the mouth corners (cheilitis)	Immune suppression or micronutrient deficiency	A gentle reminder from your body that nutrient support can restore immunity and healing
Metallic or bitter taste	Sensory disturbance or toxin/metabolite buildup	Tracking it can help catch internal imbalances, often reversible with hydration, detox or medical review
Dry, fissured or burning tongue	Dehydration or autoimmune activity	A signal to hydrate or investigate further
Discolouration (for example, dark or yellowish)	Bacterial buildup or systemic imbalance	A visual cue to address lifestyle factors or internal strain

Pay attention if you notice:

- A coating that thickens, doesn't resolve with brushing, or is accompanied by bad breath or soreness

- A tongue that appears inflamed, smooth or discoloured
- Persistent taste disturbances with no obvious cause
- Fissures, cracks or ulcerations that recur or worsen over time

Speak to a healthcare professional and let your tongue lead you towards better health.

Bad Breath or a Warning Scent?

Morning breath is common but persistent bad breath is not. We often dismiss bad breath, medically known as halitosis, usually blaming it on poor dental hygiene or the remnants of a garlicky meal. However, when halitosis becomes persistent or severe, it may serve as a potent diagnostic clue. Just as a canary in a coal mine warns of danger before it becomes visible, your breath can signal metabolic dysfunctions, infections and even life-threatening conditions before other symptoms arise.

When something smells off, look deeper

- Any ulcer or lesion that does not heal within two weeks
- Difficulty swallowing, speaking or moving the tongue
- Unexplained burning, tingling or numbness in the mouth
- Unusual swellings, persistent pain or bleeding
- Sudden change in taste or breath, particularly if associated with other symptoms like fatigue or weight loss

Stories Teeth Don't Tell Aloud

Teeth are among the hardest substances in the human body, and they are more than tools for mastication (that is, chewing). They function as forensic markers, capturing silent imprints of what your body has endured and what it may be fighting against.

Unlike skin or muscles, teeth do not regenerate. Once damaged, they carry that history forward. This makes them a biological black box, recording past traumas, ongoing deficiencies and emerging imbalances with uncanny precision.

Is Tooth Decay Just a Sugar Story?

Cavities, or dental caries, are often framed as the inevitable result of sugar, snacks and skipped brushing. And while poor oral hygiene and sugary diets are indeed major culprits, rapid, recurring or oddly located decay might be your body's way of hinting at an internal imbalance.

When teeth begin to deteriorate without an obvious cause, it's time to move beyond the toothbrush and ask: What is really eroding the enamel from within?

Fermentable Carbohydrates: While sugar is the poster child, even 'healthy' carbs like crackers, fruits and hidden sugars in packaged foods feed acid-producing oral bacteria. These bacteria create an acidic environment that softens and demineralizes enamel.

Dry Mouth (Xerostomia): Saliva is not just moisture. It neutralizes acids, washes away debris and delivers key minerals like calcium and phosphate. Common causes of reduced saliva are:

- Antidepressants, antihistamines and antihypertensives
- Autoimmune conditions like Sjögren's syndrome
- Chronic dehydration

Acid Reflux (GORD): Reflux is more than heartburn. Silent reflux can bathe the teeth in stomach acid, especially at night, wearing away the enamel over time, often starting from the back molars.

Frequent Vomiting: In conditions like bulimia nervosa, hyperemesis gravidarum (HG) and severe gastritis, the repeated exposure of teeth to gastric acid results in accelerated erosion and sensitivity.

Nutritional Deficiencies:

- Vitamin D and K2 (these are crucial for calcium absorption and regulation; without them, the enamel repair is compromised)
- Magnesium and phosphorus (key players in mineralization)
- Collagen deficiency (poor protein intake or chronic inflammation weakens the dentin beneath the enamel)

An overlooked player in tooth decay is the oral microbiome. Just like the gut, your mouth hosts a dynamic community of bacteria. A shift in this ecosystem due to antibiotics, a high-sugar diet, stress or hormonal changes can tilt the balance in favour of decay-promoting microbes like *Streptococcus mutans*.

Paying attention to your teeth could mean catching imbalances long before they manifest elsewhere in the body.

The Inflammation Link behind Gum Trouble

Your gums are not isolated tissues. They are part of a vascular, immune-integrated frontier. Changes in gum health, such as swelling or bleeding, can reflect how your body is handling inflammation overall. By paying attention to the gumline, you are not simply protecting your smile but tuning in to an important indicator of your health.

The Shaky Truth about Tooth Mobility

In childhood, a loose tooth is a celebrated milestone. In adulthood, it is a red flag that needs attention. When your teeth begin to drift, wiggle or feel unstable while chewing or brushing, it may point to issues that can result from weakening bone support, gum inflammation or imbalances in the body. Taking early signs of tooth mobility seriously can help prevent further damage and support long-term health, both dental and systemic.

Held in the Jaw, Worn on the Face

Your face is more than just the first impression you make on others. Every expression and every shift in appearance can reveal clues about what is going on inside your body. That puffiness you notice after waking up, the jaw that clicks with every bite or the sudden appearance of facial asymmetry are all signals from your body, trying to grab your attention.

So, What Is Your Face Saying?

Puffy Face: Waking up with a puffy face is not always due to too much late-night Netflix. It could be a sign of hypothyroidism (that is, an underactive thyroid) or renal issues (that is, kidney problems). Both conditions can cause fluid retention, making your face appear swollen, especially around the eyes and cheeks. If it persists, it is worth consulting your doctor.

Facial Asymmetry: A sudden droop or noticeable unevenness on one side of your face might point to Bell's palsy or even a stroke. The facial nerve controls muscle movement and when something interferes with it (whether from an infection or a blood flow issue), the face may lose its symmetry. A change in your ability to smile, blink or move your mouth on one side is a key indicator to monitor. This requires immediate attention, particularly if you also experience slurred speech or weakness in other parts of your body.

Jaw Clicking or Pain: Is your jaw making odd sounds when you chew or does it feel tender? It could be due to a problem with the temporomandibular joint (TMJ) or arthritis. Chronic jaw pain can also arise from structural issues or the overuse of the jaw muscles. Left unchecked, this discomfort can impact how you talk, eat and even breathe.

Relevance to Facial and Jaw Surgery

If you are undergoing or considering facial plastic surgery or jaw surgery, these symptoms are particularly important to watch for before and after the procedure. Surgeons will often advise monitoring for any sudden changes in the facial structure, asymmetry or discomfort to ensure the surgery's success and your recovery.

The Joker's Medical File, a Hypothetical Diagnosis

Before he became the Joker, Arthur Fleck's laughter was involuntary, his headaches were intense, and his eyes were hollow with exhaustion. The signs were there. Gotham didn't notice until it was late.

'Is it just me…or is it getting crazier out there?'

With that eerie smile and distant stare, Arthur Fleck posed a question that was less rhetorical than it was diagnostic. Beneath the greasepaint and broken laughter lay a neurological saga and a storm brewing not in society but within his own head. His skull, so often tilted with that unnerving grin, may have held neglected pathologies.

Arthur's laughter was not joy. It was sudden, jarring and painful, erupting like a short circuit through his face. His laugh bears a striking resemblance to pseudobulbar affect (PBA), which is a neurological condition caused by damage to the brainstem or associated circuits, often due to head trauma and neurodevelopmental disorders. Childhood abuse, repeated blows and oxygen deprivation could have scarred the fragile emotional regulators in his brain. Every cackle was possibly a cry masked by neurological noise.

More disturbingly, his thoughts weren't grounded in shared reality. He envisioned relationships that didn't exist, basked in imagined fame and sometimes responded to a world no one else could see. These hallucinations and delusions point towards psychosis, possibly a severe mood disorder with psychotic features. However, while his visions could be explained psychiatrically, their source may lie deeper in chemical imbalances, synaptic misfires or even frontal lobe dysfunction. The cortex, which is our seat of judgement, planning and empathy, might have been running on borrowed time.

His head bore external clues too: tremors in his jaw, erratic eye movement and that strained, stiff smile. These may indicate symptoms, potentially linked to dopamine imbalance or prolonged exposure to neurotoxins. His daily application of clown makeup using low-grade materials may have subjected him to chronic absorption of lead and cadmium (metals that are known to penetrate the blood-brain barrier and damage cognitive and motor function over time).

Arthur's condition was neuropsychiatric. His symptoms traversed disciplines. Microvascular disease, toxic exposure, trauma, inflammation: any or all might have played their part in scripting his fate.

History has seen its share of missed signals, many of which were preventable. So, awareness is vital.

The Secret Wisdom of Your Neck and Throat

Tucked within the neck's relatively compact space are some of the body's most crucial and sensitive systems: the airway that delivers every breath, the blood vessels that pump life to and from the brain, the nerves that carry commands and sensation and the vocal cords that give your voice its sound. Alongside these, the lymph nodes and thyroid gland act as early responders.

The throat, equally important, is where breathing, swallowing and speaking intersect. It is also where signs of stress, infection, inflammation and even cancer often appear first. A slight swelling, persistent hoarseness, difficulty swallowing or a chronic sore throat might seem minor, but they can sometimes signal deep-rooted issues involving the immune system, thyroid, cardiovascular system or even the brain.

In this chapter, we will decode the subtle shifts that occur in the neck and throat. What makes this region especially fascinating is how interconnected it is with daily function and systemic health.

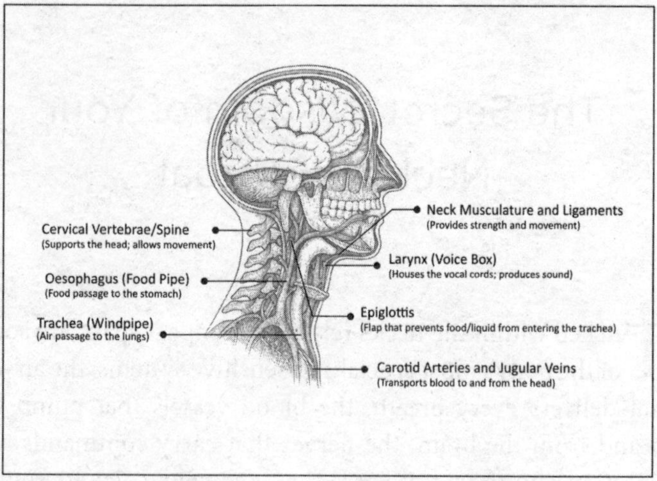

Figure 4: Anatomy of the neck and throat

Overview of Anatomy and Function

The Neck

If the human body were an ancient city, the neck would be its busiest and most guarded gateway where breath enters, blood flows, voices rise and food passes through. It is where life's essentials—that is, air, blood, voice and nutrition—must pass, uninterrupted and uncorrupted.

At a glance, the neck may appear unremarkable. But beneath the skin lies a meticulously engineered system that performs a complex balancing act every second of your life. Its primary role is deceptively simple: to support the head (which is a 4.5- to 5.5-kilogram structure that houses your brain, eyes, ears, mouth and more). Holding up this command centre requires coordinated strength and fine-tuned balance, especially as your head moves in multiple directions, sometimes rapidly or unpredictably.

The Throat

The throat is one of the only places in the human body where two vital but conflicting life processes (that is, breathing and eating) must take turns without ever colliding. And yet, they do so in milliseconds, thousands of times a day, often without conscious thought, ensuring that food goes down the oesophagus while air flows into the trachea and never the other way around. This feat is orchestrated by a small flap called the epiglottis, which acts like a bouncer at the throat's club (snapping shut over the windpipe every time you swallow, only to reopen for the next breath).

This balancing act is delicate. One misfire—due to distraction, neurological dysfunction, age-related slowing or even simple exhaustion—and the consequences may be immediate and terrifying. That's when food or liquid 'goes down the wrong pipe,' triggering a violent coughing fit. In severe cases, it may lead to aspiration, choking or even silent pneumonia, especially in the elderly and those with neuromuscular disorders.

The throat is also your instrument of expression. Inside it lies the larynx, or voice box, where your pitch, tone and every emotional nuance of your voice, from laughter to lament, is shaped. Even your first cry as a newborn, which is the primal declaration of life, passes through this gateway.

Further, each person's voice is as unique as a fingerprint, thanks to differences in vocal cord size, tension and shape. Even identical twins have distinct voices.

As we move forward, you will learn how to listen with intent, recognize the body's early alarms, understand their causes and intervene before the quiet becomes chaos. Because in the world of preventive health, even the smallest sensation is worth listening to.

Neck Pain and Stiffness

Neck pain is one of the most frequently reported musculoskeletal complaints in the modern world, affecting millions across all age groups.[7] It often begins subtly in the form of a stiff morning neck and a dull ache by evening, and it can quickly escalate into debilitating discomfort that restricts movement, sleep and function.

Muscular Causes: In most cases, neck pain arises from muscle strain or tension, especially in people who spend long hours at a desk (hunched over screens) or drive for extended periods. Stress, too, has a direct link with neck pain. When you are anxious or overwhelmed, your body often responds by clenching muscles, especially around the neck and shoulders. Another common cause is whiplash, which is an injury resulting from a sudden, forceful movement of the head, usually backward and then forward as in car accidents.

Nerve-Related Causes: When the pain radiates into the shoulders, arms and hands or is accompanied by numbness, tingling and weakness, it may be nerve-related. Common causes include: herniated (slipped/ruptured) discs pressing

---

[7]Hoy, Damian, Lyn March, Anthony Woolf, Fiona Blyth, Peter Brooks, Emma Smith, Theo Vos, Jan Barendregt, Jed Blore, Chris Murray, Roy Burstein, and Rachelle Buchbinder, 'The Global Burden of Neck Pain: Estimates from the Global Burden of Disease 2010 Study', *Annals of the Rheumatic Diseases*, Vol. 73, No. 7, 2014, pp. 1309–15, https://doi.org/10.1136/annrheumdis-2013-204431. Accessed on 8 December 2025.

on nerves, bone spurs from ageing joints and degenerative disc disease.

Joint-Related Pain: The joints of the cervical spine are common sources of neck pain. With age or overuse, cartilage can wear down, leading to stiffness, pain, reduced motion and sometimes a grinding sound (called crepitus) when turning the head. Osteoarthritis can also affect these joints, causing inflammation and bony growths that may press on nerves or limit movement.

When Neck Pain Is a Medical Emergency

While most neck pain is benign and self-limiting, certain features warrant immediate medical attention:

Fever, Headache and Neck Stiffness: These symptoms may indicate meningitis, which is a potentially life-threatening infection of the brain and spinal cord coverings. While rare, it is wise to consult a doctor if they appear together and persist.

Sudden Severe Pain after Injury: If sharp neck pain follows a fall or accident, it might indicate something more than a strain, such as spinal instability or a small fracture. Medical evaluation can help rule out anything serious.

Neurological Symptoms: Unusual symptoms like limb weakness, balance issues or bladder changes may be linked to nerve compression in the spine. These signs don't always mean serious trouble, but early medical input helps ensure the right care.

Always treat unexplained, worsening or persistent neck pain seriously.

What Neck Swelling Really Means

The neck houses over 300 lymph nodes, which are part of the immune system's surveillance network. These nodes filter fluid, trap pathogens and raise an alarm when needed. Most commonly, lymph nodes swell in response to infections:

- Viral (like mononucleosis, HIV and common colds)
- Bacterial (strep throat, dental abscesses and infected wounds)
- Tuberculosis (a cause of slow-growing, sometimes painless lymph node enlargement)

These nodes are typically tender and mobile and decrease in size once the infection resolves. However, lumps that are painless, hard or fixed and continue growing over weeks may suggest something more serious, such as:

- Lymphoma (a cancer of the lymphatic system)
- Metastatic cancers (from the mouth, throat, thyroid or even breast and lungs)
- Thyroid malignancies (especially if associated with voice changes and difficulty swallowing)

A single unexplained lump persisting for more than three weeks should not be ignored. Early evaluation is important.

Not Every Sore Throat Is 'Just a Cold'

Perhaps the most common complaint, a sore throat can stem from numerous causes. Most often, it is due to viral infections like the common cold, influenza and COVID-19. These are usually self-limiting, accompanied by fever, fatigue and nasal congestion.

But some sore throats are bacterial, such as strep throat and tonsillitis. These can lead to complications like rheumatic fever and kidney inflammation if untreated. Clues include:

- Severe pain
- Swollen tonsils with white patches
- High fever
- Painful lymph nodes

Allergies, dry air and even irritants like cigarette smoke can also inflame the throat. Chronic sore throats may indicate acid reflux, especially in people who experience burning in the chest or a sour taste.

Hoarseness and Voice Changes

Your voice is produced by the vocal cords in the voice box, and changes here can be very revealing. Hoarseness may result from:

- Laryngitis (often viral or post-infectious)
- Vocal cord strain from overuse
- Reflux laryngitis, where acid irritates the cords
- Nodules or polyps in professional voice users

Persistent hoarseness, especially in smokers and individuals over 40, should not be ignored, particularly if it is accompanied by weight loss, throat discomfort or trouble swallowing. While often harmless, it may signal something more serious in some cases, like laryngeal cancer, and early evaluation can make all the difference.

Difficulty in Swallowing

Swallowing should be effortless. When it isn't, there may be a range of causes:

- Neurological (stroke, Parkinson's or motor neurone disease that can affect muscle coordination)
- Structural (enlarged tonsils, tumours or oesophageal strictures that can block the passage)
- Muscular (conditions like myasthenia gravis or muscular dystrophy that can weaken the swallow)

Choking, coughing during meals and unintentional weight loss are signs that deserve timely medical attention. While they may have simple causes, it is best to rule out anything more serious early on.

Thyroid-Related Alarms

Hyperthyroidism (When the Body Is in Overdrive)

When the thyroid becomes overactive, it releases an excess of hormones that push the body into a hyper-alert state. People may lose weight despite a healthy or even increased appetite, experience a racing heart, shaky hands or anxious moods, and feel persistently warm or sweaty. Sometimes, the neck swells visibly.

The most common cause is Graves' disease. It is an autoimmune disorder where the body's own antibodies overstimulate the thyroid. Left unmanaged, this condition can disrupt heart rhythms and, in rare cases, trigger a dangerous escalation known as a thyroid storm.

Hypothyroidism (When the Body Slows Down)

An underactive thyroid can bring the body into a low gear. Energy levels dip, weight creeps up and even a slight chill feels unbearable. People may feel unusually down or mentally foggy, while changes in skin texture, hair health, facial puffiness and voice hoarseness can also appear.

The most common culprit is Hashimoto's thyroiditis. It is an autoimmune disorder where the immune system mistakenly targets the thyroid, gradually wearing down its function.

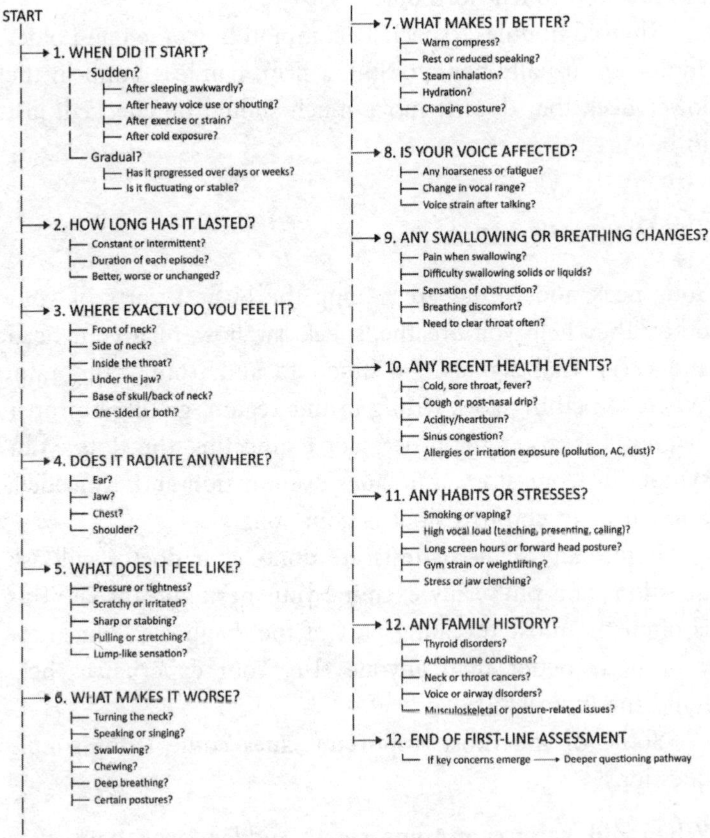

Figure 5: *The diagnostic lens*

Goitre and Nodules

An enlarged thyroid, or goitre, may appear as a smooth swelling or a lumpy cluster in the neck. While most goitres are harmless and often go unnoticed, some can affect swallowing or breathing if they grow large enough, or they may occasionally produce too much hormone.

Thyroid nodules, especially common in women and older adults, are usually benign. Still, a firm, painless lump in the lower neck that doesn't move much should be checked, just to be sure.

The Diagnostic Lens

Your neck and throat are among the busiest parts of your body. They help you breathe, speak, swallow, turn your head and carry vital signals and blood to and from your brain. When something goes wrong in this region, getting a proper diagnosis is a careful process of connecting the dots: your symptoms, your story, a doctor's examination and, if needed, a few tests to confirm what is going on.

Before any scans or tests are done, your doctor will ask questions and physically examine your neck and throat. This is often the most revealing part of the diagnosis. You know your body better than anyone else. Your experiences help build the first picture.

Some of the most important clues come from simple questions:

When did your symptoms start? Sudden neck pain after sleeping awkwardly is different from a slow-growing lump that's been there for months.

How long have they lasted? Something that comes and goes may be less serious than something that gets worse over time.

What else is happening? A sore throat with a fever may point to an infection. A lump with unexplained weight loss might be something more serious.

Other questions may include whether you smoke, drink, use your voice a lot or have family members with similar issues. All of this helps narrow down possible causes.

Next, your doctor will examine your neck and throat. They will check for lumps, swelling and tenderness. The thyroid gland, lymph nodes and muscles are all gently examined. You may be asked to turn or tilt your head to see if movement is stiff or painful. Further, a simple look at your tonsils, tongue and back of the throat can reveal redness, swelling, pus or other signs of infection or irritation.

This hands-on approach often gives the doctor a strong sense of what is going on, sometimes enough to diagnose and treat right away.

How to Care for Your Neck and Throat

The colossal necks of dinosaurs like the Brachiosaurus weren't built for reach only. They were survival machines in the form of towering sensors that scanned the world for threat or opportunity. In evolution, height meant foresight. Strangely, your own neck serves a similar purpose, as it quietly senses shifts within.

Caring for this region begins with posture. When your head is tilted forward, even slightly, your neck bears the burden of several extra kilos. That strain builds silently, often leading to pain, stiffness and nerve issues. Keeping screens at eye level, avoiding awkward sleeping positions and sitting with your head stacked above your spine can undo more damage than you might imagine.

Your throat, meanwhile, thrives on hydration. Dryness, on the other hand, is an invitation for irritation, infections and even voice issues. Sip water regularly, especially if you are in air-conditioned rooms, and give your vocal cords a break when they feel strained. Whispering, surprisingly, can hurt more than help. Speak gently, instead.

And then, there is stress. It tightens your neck, clenches your jaw and can leave you with that 'lump in the throat' feeling that seems to have no cause. Unwind often. Stretch. Breathe. Move.

The real care lies in learning how to listen.

Shoulders Bear the Weight, Arms Bridge the Gap, Hands Build the Future

Healthy hands move without hesitation. Arms stretch, lift, hold and embrace without complaint. Shoulders roll back with ease, rather than effort. There is no swelling, no tingling and no unexplained fatigue. There is just a seamless function, the kind you only notice when it is gone. When your joints aren't stiff, your nerves aren't screaming and your grip doesn't fail you mid-coffee—it's health humming in the background.

Think of it like owning a well-tuned wand. You flick, and it works. No misfires, no sparks and no unexpected jelly-legs. Unless, of course, you are 'Ron Weasley.'

Pain Is Not Random

When your right shoulder stiffens for no apparent reason, your left arm begins to throb unprovoked and your fingers swell or your grip weakens, it is not a coincidence. It is a coded message that only the body knows how to deliver and only the observant knows how to decode.

Consider the shoulder, which is a marvel of mobility and complexity. It offers more movement than almost any other joint in the human body. However, with this mobility comes vulnerability. While rotator cuff injuries and musculoskeletal strain are common causes behind shoulder discomfort, it's worth remembering that pain in this region isn't always orthopaedic in nature. Sometimes, persistent tension may reflect chronic emotional stress, subtly shaping posture and muscle tone over time.

In rare cases, shoulder pain, especially on the left side, can even be a referred sign of cardiac distress. Though such instances are uncommon, they remind us that the body communicates in layered ways.

Now, move downward. The arms are strong and sturdy, but even strength can falter in subtle ways. A tingling forearm, a creeping numbness or an unexpected heaviness when reaching overhead may simply reflect poor posture or muscle fatigue. And most often, they do. However, on occasion, such sensations can hint at deeper concerns, like nerve compression, vascular changes or even early signs of neurological or cardiovascular conditions.

Then, there are the hands. A slight tremor can rattle a surgeon's confidence and a stiff joint can pause an artist mid-stroke. While most hand discomforts are minor or temporary, certain patterns like persistent swelling, numbness, stiffness or unusual cold sensitivity can be early signs of underlying conditions such as rheumatoid arthritis, diabetes, thyroid imbalances or neurological disorders. These signs rarely appear without context and often unfold gradually. A dropped pen, a fumbled button or a sharp reaction to cold, for instance, may seem trivial but can be subtle alarms.

Not every signal is urgent, yet each one deserves some attention.

This chapter does not ask you to overanalyse every

sensation. It demands something harder: awareness. The kind that can tell the difference between a harmless twitch and a herald of something graver.

The Shoulders

In the magical world of Harry Potter, the shoulders of each character carry more than their cloaks and wands. Harry's own shoulders, for example, bear the unbearable weight of destiny, loss and relentless responsibility even as a boy. Hermione Granger's stoop, often from hunching over heavy books, is not just a physical posture but also reflects the burden of perfectionism, intellect and a deep sense of social responsibility. And Ron Weasley? His drooping shoulders often echo feelings of inadequacy and of living in the shadows of others despite his courage.

Thus, even in fiction, shoulders are rarely just bones and joints. And in real life, they are no different.

Structurally, the shoulder joint is a miracle of motion. It is the most mobile joint in the human body, allowing for an astonishing range of movement (up, down, forward, backward and all the way around). However, with that freedom comes a price. The shoulder's very design makes it vulnerable to dislocation, strain, impingement and injury.

At the core of thc shoulder complex are the glenohumeral joint, where the upper arm meets the shoulder blade; the rotator cuff, which stabilizes movement; the scapula or shoulder blade; and the clavicle, or collarbone. If even one element falters through injury, overuse or systemic disease, the entire mechanism suffers.

The Posture Effect

Walk into any office, and you will see it: the hunched shoulders, the forward neck and the rounded back. Poor posture doesn't just look tired, but it also feels tired. It reduces lung capacity, affects digestion, creates muscular imbalances and, over time, contributes to chronic pain.

Good posture is less about sitting rigidly and more about dynamic alignment. Move often. Sit upright with your ears aligned over your shoulders. Adjust the screens to eye level. Support your lower back. And most importantly, stretch the chest while strengthening the upper back, correcting the muscular imbalances that poor posture creates.

The Frozen Shoulder

There are few sensations more frustrating than realizing that your own arm refuses to obey. Frozen shoulder, or adhesive capsulitis, creeps in silently. What begins as a mild ache hardens into stiffness so severe that even basic tasks like reaching overhead and dressing become a daily struggle. In this condition, the capsule surrounding your shoulder joint becomes inflamed and thickened, forming adhesions that restrict movement. It is like your shoulder has been slowly welded into place.

Frozen shoulder commonly affects people over forty, particularly women, and is strongly associated with:

- Diabetes (Type 1 or 2)
- Thyroid disorders
- Periods of immobility (post-surgery, injury or illness)
- Autoimmune conditions

The earlier the frozen shoulder is diagnosed, the better the outcome. Left alone, the shoulder may improve on its own, but at a glacial pace.

The Rotator Cuff Dilemma

Imagine trying to comb your hair, reach a shelf or simply lift a teacup, only to be halted by a sharp, lingering pain in your shoulder. This is often the daily reality for those suffering from rotator cuff injuries, an extremely common yet frequently underestimated issue.

The rotator cuff is a group of four muscles and their tendons that stabilize the shoulder and allow it to move in multiple directions. When this structure is injured, even the smallest motion can become a painful ordeal. Two of the most prevalent issues affecting the rotator cuff are:

Rotator Cuff Tendinopathy: A degeneration or inflammation of the tendons due to overuse or age-related wear

Rotator Cuff Tears: Partial or complete ruptures of one or more tendons, often due to trauma, repetitive strain or degeneration

These conditions are most commonly seen in:

- Athletes, particularly those involved in throwing sports, swimming and tennis
- Manual labourers, whose work demands repetitive shoulder motion and heavy lifting
- Older adults, as the tendons naturally weaken and degenerate with age

Addressed early, most cases respond well to therapy, medical management or, when necessary, surgical repair.

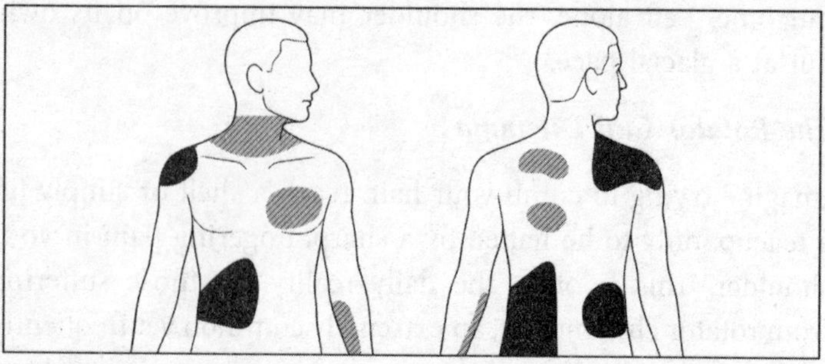

HEART	GALLBLADDER
• Centre and left side of the chest • Left side of the neck and throat • Left shoulder • Inner side of the left arm and forearm • Upper back between the shoulder blades	• Right upper abdomen • Right lower chest / right costal margin • Right shoulder • Right side of the upper back, below the shoulder blade

Figure 6: Hidden causes of shoulder pain

Referred Pain from the Heart or Gallbladder

One of the most overlooked causes of shoulder pain is the heart.

A dull, deep or pressure-like pain in the left shoulder, especially when it arises suddenly and without apparent cause, can be a sign of cardiac ischaemia (that is, insufficient blood flow to the heart muscle) or even a myocardial infarction (that is, heart attack). This referred pain often travels through shared nerve pathways, particularly via the spinal cord segments that serve both the heart and shoulder (C5–T1). The brain, unable to distinguish the source clearly, interprets the distress as shoulder pain.

This is why symptoms of a heart attack can include:

- Discomfort or heaviness in the left shoulder or arm
- Tightness or pressure in the chest

- Jaw or upper back pain
- Sweating, shortness of breath, nausea and a sense of unease

These signs may be subtle, particularly in women, older adults and people with diabetes, and are often mistaken for muscle strain, indigestion and anxiety. Nonetheless, any unexplained upper body discomfort, especially if accompanied by systemic symptoms, warrants immediate evaluation.

On the opposite side of the body lies another master of disguise: the gallbladder.

When inflamed or infected (a condition known as cholecystitis), the gallbladder may refer pain to the right shoulder or shoulder blade. Signs of gallbladder-related referred shoulder pain often include:

- Sharp or cramping pain in the upper right abdomen
- Pain radiating to the right shoulder or between the shoulder blades
- Bloating, nausea and vomiting, particularly after eating fatty meals
- Tenderness in the right upper quadrant upon touch

So, if your shoulder pain is persistent and one-sided, particularly on the left, which may occasionally signal cardiac issues, or on the right, which can sometimes reflect gallbladder involvement, it is worth paying attention to it. While most shoulder pain is musculoskeletal, symptoms that are unusual, severe or accompanied by other signs should prompt timely medical evaluation.

Unlike mechanical shoulder pain, which typically worsens with movement, referred pain is often unaffected by shoulder activity, and that's a key distinction.

MRI	X-Ray	CT Scan
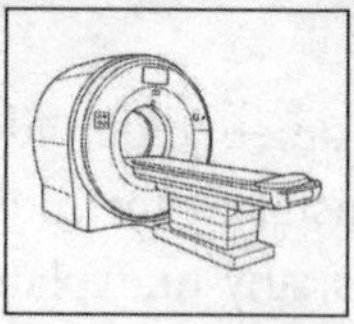	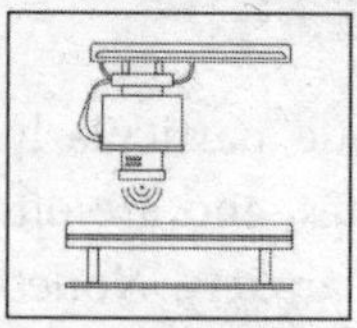	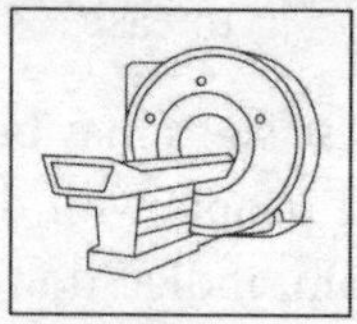
Used to evaluate soft tissues, brain, spine, joints and internal organs	Used to evaluate bones, chest and lungs, and to detect fractures or infections	Used to evaluate bones, organs and blood vessels, and to detect injuries or disease
Remove all metal, such as jewellery, watches, hairpins and cards, and inform staff about implants or past surgeries	Remove metal in the area being scanned, with no special preparation usually needed	Remove metal near the scan area and follow instructions if contrast is used; fasting may be required
No radiation; the strong magnet can attract metal objects, and all metal must be removed before entering the room	Uses X-ray radiation; limit exposure and use shielding when possible	Uses higher radiation than X-rays; only perform scans when medically necessary
Gadolinium contrast may be used; inform staff of kidney problems, prior allergic reactions or pregnancy	Contrast is rarely needed; usually safe without it	Iodine-based contrast may be used; disclose kidney problems, allergies or asthma
Machine is loud; wear ear protection, stay very still, and some people may feel claustrophobic	Quick and quiet; stay still briefly	Short scan; may feel enclosed, stay still, and staff monitors throughout

Figure 7: Differences among MRI, X-ray and CT scan

The Emotional Shoulder

Have you ever observed someone gripped by anxiety? Their brow furrows, their fists clench, and almost without fail, their shoulders rise. It's as if the body is bracing itself for an invisible blow. The phenomenon is well-documented in both neuroscience and somatic psychology.[8] The trapezius

[8]Porges, Stephen W., 'The Polyvagal Theory: New Insights into Adaptive Reactions of the Autonomic Nervous System', *Cleveland Clinic Journal of Medicine,*' Vol. 76, Suppl. 2, 2009, pp. S86–S90, https://doi.org/10.3949/ccjm.76.s2.17. Accessed on 8 December 2025; Ogden, Pat, Kekuni Minton, and Clare Pain, *Trauma and the Body: A Sensorimotor Approach to Psychotherapy,* W.W. Norton & Company, New York, 2006.

muscles, especially the upper fibres that span from the neck to the shoulders, are highly responsive to chronic stress. They tighten subtly at first, holding all the tension, and over time, the stiffness becomes a part of one's posture, one's gait and even one's identity.

This form of pain or tightness is insidious because it often eludes detection. You can scan the area with an X-ray or MRI and find nothing wrong, yet the discomfort is real.

Modern life, with its relentless pace and digital demands, fuels this state of shoulder hypervigilance. Hours spent hunched over a computer or phone, coupled with emotional pressure, create a perfect storm. The body doesn't know you are just replying to emails. It reacts as though it is under attack. And the shoulders respond, again and again, by bracing, tightening and holding.

Left unchecked, this emotional tension can evolve into:

- Chronic myofascial pain
- Tension headaches
- Reduced shoulder mobility
- And a persistent feeling of being physically and emotionally 'wound up'

So, what can be done when stress chooses the shoulders as its nesting ground?

The truth is, your shoulders remember what your mind tries to forget. They hold every sigh stifled, every confrontation avoided and every burden borne in silence.

Listen to their tension. It is a form of self-care and inner respect.

The Arms

There is something profoundly human about allowing someone to fall asleep on your arm. It is not just about physical proximity but it is also about trust, sacrifice and care bundled into one quiet gesture. You bear their weight, even as your own arm begins to tingle or ache, refusing to move for fear of disturbing their peace. The arm becomes more than a limb. And still, while we extend our arms in affection, comfort and protection, how often do we listen to them in return?

Arms are expressive. We raise them to cheer, stretch them when tired, fold them in contemplation and reach out with them when in need. They house some of the most vital nerves, muscles and blood vessels of the upper body. And when something goes wrong, be it neurological, circulatory or musculoskeletal, our arms signal.

Unfortunately, the challenge is that we often misread those signals or dismiss them entirely.

In the pages ahead, we will uncover the early murmurs of serious conditions and the invisible alarms cloaked in everyday sensations. So, consider this a pact between you and your body. Before you offer your arms again as a place of peace for someone else, make sure they are not crying out beneath the silence.

When Tingling Isn't Just a Tingle

We have all experienced that pins-and-needles feeling when we have slept awkwardly or leaned on an arm too long. It is usually harmless and passes quickly. But what if it doesn't? Persistent tingling, numbness and burning sensations in the arms can indicate a range of underlying issues:

Peripheral Neuropathy: Often caused by diabetes, this may begin with subtle tingling in the hands and forearms, especially at night.

Cervical Radiculopathy: This results from nerve root compression in the neck (yes, this is the one overlap with shoulders), leading to shooting pain or electric shock-like sensations radiating down the arm.

Carpal Tunnel Syndrome: This is typically associated with the hands, often starting with tingling that moves up the forearm, especially during sleep.

Here is a helpful distinction: If tingling wakes you up at night, affects both hands symmetrically and improves by shaking your hands out, think carpal tunnel. If it follows a distinct nerve path from the neck down one arm, suspect a cervical cause. And if it starts subtly in both arms and worsens gradually, particularly in diabetics, consider peripheral neuropathy.

In all cases, persistent numbness or tingling shouldn't be brushed off. It may be your nervous system's way of asking for attention.

The Disappearing Act of Muscle Power

The strength of the human arm is astonishing, being capable of holding, lifting, throwing and restraining. So, when you begin to notice a cup feels heavier than it should or that bags strain you more than before, take note. Unexplained weakness in the arms, particularly when it is one-sided or progressive, can hint at early motor neurone diseases, brachial plexus injuries from trauma or sleep posture, or even multiple sclerosis when paired with vision or balance issues.

What's crucial here is the pattern. Temporary fatigue from

exertion is one thing. However, the weakness that doesn't improve with rest or seems to be creeping in, day by day, demands attention. If your arm tires faster than the rest of your body or starts 'misbehaving' (that is, dropping things, shaking and struggling), don't ignore the signs.

When That Arm Ache Isn't Just a Workout Thing

Arm pain, unless you have just returned from the gym, should be treated with suspicion, especially if it is not directly linked to physical exertion.

The most dangerous form of arm pain? The kind associated with the heart. Left arm pain, especially if dull, radiating or accompanied by shortness of breath, jaw discomfort or cold sweats, may indicate a cardiac event. It doesn't always have to be crushing chest pain. In women and diabetics, heart attacks often masquerade as vague upper body discomfort, including in the arms, as mentioned earlier.

Right arm pain, though less classically associated with the heart, can also indicate systemic issues, particularly gallbladder disease or liver congestion in rare cases.

If your arm pain appears suddenly, worsens with activity and accompanies other systemic symptoms, it deserves urgent evaluation.

The Language of the Arm's Skin

Your arms can also reflect what's going on internally through their colour, texture and temperature. So, watch for changes in colour, temperature and texture as they can be important alarms too.

Bluish or purplish discolouration (cyanosis)	A hint that oxygen delivery may be reduced or that circulation is not flowing as it should
Pale, cold arms	Could reflect narrowed arteries or a reactive vessel response as seen in Raynaud's
Sudden redness, warmth and swelling (especially one-sided)	May point to a clot deep within the vein, which is a condition that calls for immediate attention
Brown patches or staining on the forearms	Often a trace of long-standing circulation issues, where blood pigments settle in the skin

Changes in skin colour, when paired with symptoms like pain, fatigue and swelling, should prompt immediate medical review. Subtle shifts in tone or texture can offer early alarms that shouldn't be overlooked.

What's That Shiver under Your Skin?

We have all experienced that sudden, fluttering movement under the skin, like a trapped moth beating its wings. A twitch in the bicep after a strenuous workout. A flicker in the upper arm following a day of poor sleep and too much caffeine. These are called muscle fasciculations (that is, tiny, involuntary contractions of the muscle fibres) and they are surprisingly common.

While occasional twitches are typically harmless, persistent or unexplained fasciculations can sometimes signal early dysfunction in the motor neurons, which are critical nerve cells responsible for sending signals from the brain to the muscles.

So, it is important to watch for accompanying warning signs, which may include:

- Twitches with weakness and muscle thinning
- Cramping or stiffness in the arms
- Worsening fatigue over time

When the Arms Feel 'Heavy' Emotionally

Yes, emotional burden can show up even in the arms. People undergoing depression or anxiety often report a sense of heaviness or numbness in the upper limbs. It's as if the weight of their thoughts is distributed into their extremities. In some, this even mimics cardiac symptoms, leading to what is termed 'non-cardiac chest pain' with referred sensations in the arms.

While the pain isn't imaginary, its roots lie in the nervous system's complex interaction with emotional centres in the brain. It is essential to acknowledge such discomfort as legitimate and treat it holistically through therapy, mindfulness and sometimes medication.

The Hands

When we marry, we seal the promise not with words alone but with a ring, placed gently on the fourth finger of the hand. The hand. It is through the hands that we swear allegiance, make vows and forge bonds. They are witnesses to our most sacred moments and also our darkest ones.

Anatomically, each hand is a marvel: 27 bones, 34 muscles, over 100 ligaments and a dense forest of nerves. These nerves do not merely allow for dexterity but they also connect to the spine and brain like copper wires to a fuse box. Blood vessels thread through the hand like rivers feeding farmland. Disrupt one and the crop fails. Interfere with the nerve and the power flickers. Block the blood flow and frost creeps in, sometimes literally.

The hand is the only place where skin, bone, tendon, nerve and vessel all lie close to the surface, exposed and visible. That's why it becomes such an accurate early-warning system.

The Mystery behind Hand Tremors

Hand tremors are among the most theatrical signs that the nervous system offers. And while the casual observer may see only a twitch, the trained eye recognizes a potential prelude to a larger story. Some tremors are entirely physiological (common during moments of emotional stress, physical exhaustion and hunger). These are transient and benign and require no deeper scrutiny. However, others bear the fingerprints of malfunction and can be usually attributed to:

Parkinson's Disease

- Starts with a resting tremor, usually in one hand
- Appears when the hand is relaxed, not while reaching or moving
- May feel like a rhythmic 'pill-rolling' motion between the thumb and forefinger
- Progresses gradually, and is often accompanied by slowness, stiffness and changes in handwriting

Essential Tremor

- A movement-based tremor, often affecting both hands
- Becomes evident during tasks like eating, writing and using utensils
- Can run in families and often worsens with age

- Not life-threatening, but it significantly affects quality of life

Hyperthyroidism

- Causes a fine, rapid tremor in the hands
- Usually accompanied by weight loss, palpitations and anxiety
- Due to overstimulation of the nervous system by excess thyroid hormone

Hypoglycaemia in Diabetics

- Sudden hand tremors paired with confusion, sweating and dizziness
- A cry for glucose (immediate sugar intake is life-saving)

Medication-Induced Tremors

- Certain drugs like bronchodilators, antidepressants and antiepileptics may cause or worsen tremors

Each of these tremors is telling a different tale: neurological, metabolic, emotional and even pharmaceutical. The key is to notice when the body stutters and ask why.

Why Do Your Hands Hurt? Let's Talk Joint Pain

It often starts quietly: an ache when you twist a bottle cap, a stiffness in the morning that makes it hard to grip your toothbrush, a dull pain that seems to come and go with the weather. Many write it off as 'just getting older,' as if that alone should excuse discomfort and as if pain is a price we are supposed to pay for time.

However, joint pain, especially in the hands, is rarely without meaning. For many, the cause is osteoarthritis (which is the slow erosion of cartilage that cushions the joints). It is more common as we age, particularly in women after menopause. The signs are gradual but persistent:

- Pain that worsens with use
- Stiffness after inactivity, easing once you get moving
- A grinding sensation as though the bones are speaking directly to you
- The appearance of bony lumps on the fingers (Heberden's and Bouchard's nodes)

However, not all joint pain is wear and tear. In some cases, it may signal an underlying inflammatory or autoimmune condition. See a doctor, ideally a rheumatologist, for proper testing: bloodwork, imaging and a detailed history. Start your treatment early, for the goal is to preserve movement and prevent long-term damage.

Not Just Pins and Needles

It often begins at night. A tingling in the thumb, index and middle fingers. A numbness that wakes you. You shake your hand vigorously and the feeling returns, for now. But over weeks or months, the reprieve shortens. Dropping objects becomes frequent. Typing becomes torturous.

Carpal tunnel syndrome (CTS) is among the most common and under-addressed conditions affecting the hand. It results from compression of the median nerve as it travels through the narrow carpal tunnel at the wrist. Repetitive motion workers, writers, assembly line workers, cashiers, musicians, pregnant women and those with diabetes or thyroid issues—the list of those at risk is broad. And contrary to popular belief, computer use is only a partial contributor. Inflammatory states that cause tissue swelling often play a greater role.

If left unmanaged, carpal tunnel syndrome (CTS) can lead to long-term nerve damage. Nonetheless, with timely diagnosis and the right treatment, most people experience significant relief and can return to normal function without lasting effects.

Wellness at Your Fingertips

The shoulders, arms and hands are the instruments of creation and destruction, as well as of grace and grit. With them, we wage wars, write laws, comfort children, compose sonatas and sign away empires. From the earliest cave etchings to the last text message, the shoulders, arms and hands have been our agents of intent.

So, pause. Take notice!

What are your hands doing when you are not thinking about them? Are your shoulders quietly holding tension? Are your arms tired before your day even ends? Do your wrists crack a little too often or do your fingers tingle when they rest?

We often focus on the big picture, involving our heart, brain or gut health, while forgetting the joints and nerves that move us through the world every single day. However, the truth is, dysfunction in the upper limbs can affect everything from how we work to how we express ourselves, how we sleep, how we hug and even how we heal.

So, shrug off the stiffness. Roll those shoulders like you are dancing in secret. Give your wrists a break. And keep those fingers moving.

The Power Pose

You have likely heard of the 'power pose': standing tall, chest out, shoulders back and hands placed on your hips. It is a simple stance, but studies have shown that adopting such a posture can boost feelings of confidence and power.[9] It is a physical representation of strength, where the chest and upper back form the core of the body's frame and project not just physical presence but mental fortitude. This pose taps into the body's alignment, setting a tone for how we interact with the world around us. The open chest signifies openness and strength while the strong back gives us balance and stability.

Having said that, this 'power pose' isn't just about looking confident. It is also about feeling confident internally. The chest, the heart and the lungs are intricately linked to our sense of self. When our chest is open, we breathe freely, our heart beats steadily and our spirit feels unburdened. A strong, aligned upper back supports this function by keeping our

---

[9]Carney, Dana R., Amy J.C. Cuddy, and Andy J. Yap, 'Power Posing: Brief Nonverbal Displays Affect Neuroendocrine Levels and Risk Tolerance', *Psychological Science*, Vol. 21, No. 10, 2010, pp. 1363–68, https://doi.org/10.1177/0956797610383437; Ranehill, Eva, Anna Dreber, Magnus Johannesson, Susanne Leiberg, Sunhae Sul, and Roberto A. Weber, 'Assessing the Robustness of Power Posing: No Effect on Hormones and Risk Tolerance in a Large Sample of Men and Women', *Psychological Science*, Vol. 26, No. 5, 2015, pp. 653–56, https://doi.org/10.1177/0956797614553946. Both accessed on 8 December 2025.

spine in place, offering the stability needed for clear posture and movement.

Together, the chest and upper back create a sense of strength and presence that is as much about internal harmony as it is about outward projection.

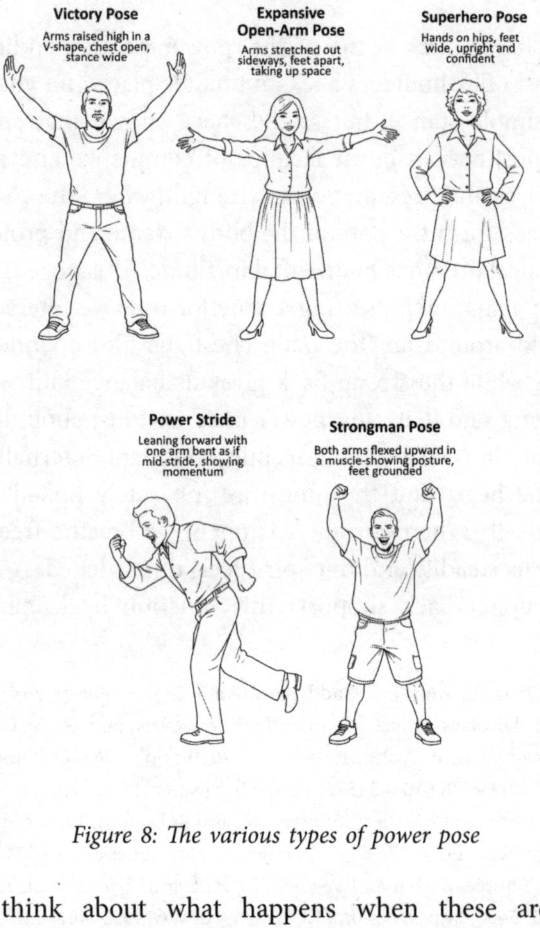
Victory Pose
Arms raised high in a V-shape, chest open, stance wide
Expansive Open-Arm Pose
Arms stretched out sideways, feet apart, taking up space
Superhero Pose
Hands on hips, feet wide, upright and confident
Power Stride
Leaning forward with one arm bent as if mid-stride, showing momentum
Strongman Pose
Both arms flexed upward in a muscle-showing posture, feet grounded

Figure 8: The various types of power pose

Now, think about what happens when these areas are compromised (when the chest becomes tight, the back weakens or the posture gives way). Suddenly, that sense of strength evaporates. Breathing becomes shallow, the body feels restricted and the mind follows suit. Tension in the chest and upper back manifests physically as well as emotionally, creating a cycle of discomfort that erodes both our physical and emotional well-being.

The Chest and Upper Back Chronicles

Deep-sea researchers have long studied a peculiar phenomenon: Certain fish, when brought to the surface too quickly, don't bleed or thrash.[10] *Instead, the rapid change in pressure causes the gas in their swim bladders and tissues to expand, leading to barotrauma, damaging their bodies without external signs.*

The organs housed within the chest are essential to our survival and yet it is here that some of the most critical and life-changing alarms originate. A slight irregularity in the beating heart, a brief catch in the breath or a subtle change in the way we feel can be signs of a deeper issue that demands attention. Perhaps, it's as startling as the fact that a heart attack can occur without chest pain. Some individuals experience what is known as a 'silent heart attack,' where the only signs can be mild dizziness, fatigue or discomfort in the jaw or shoulder. This phenomenon is particularly dangerous because it often goes undetected until significant damage has been done.

The lungs, too, hold alarms that are easily overlooked. For instance, a persistent cough that lasts more than three

---

[10]Kerr, J.R., P.R. White, T.G. Leighton, L.G.M. Silva, and P.S. Kemp, 'Boyle's Law Ignores Dynamic Processes in Governing Barotrauma in Fish,' *Scientific Reports*, Vol. 13, No. 1, 2023, Article no. 19125, https://doi.org/10.1038/s41598-023-46125-9. Accessed on 10 December 2025.

weeks can be a sign of something as serious as lung cancer or tuberculosis, but many people dismiss it as the common cold that simply won't go away. Asthma, a condition that affects nearly 350 million people worldwide, can also be insidious in its onset, with sufferers sometimes unaware that they are slowly losing the ability to breathe fully.[11] These subtle signals are all part of the body's complex warning system, and yet we often disregard them in the rush of daily life.

Further, did you know that chronic upper back pain can actually contribute to issues in the neck, shoulders and even the hips, leading to a cascade of musculoskeletal problems? This is because the upper back, specifically the thoracic spine, acts as the body's central pivot. It's no surprise, then, that 80% of people are likely to experience upper back pain in their lifetime, often linked to poor posture, repetitive strain and stress.[12]

This chapter is your guided reconnaissance of the chest and upper back, where body alarms may either sound like thunder or whisper like fog. By learning to tune in to the early warnings of discomfort, strain or pain in these vital areas, we can better protect our health.

Is It the Heart or the Frame?

A sudden ache in the chest can feel like an instinctive jolt that something may be deeply wrong. Rightly so. Chest pain is among the body's most alarming signals, but not every

---

[11]Enilari, Oladunni, and Sumita Sinha, 'The Global Impact of Asthma in Adult Populations', *Annals of Global Health*, Vol. 85, No. 1, 2019, p. 2, https://doi.org/10.5334/aogh.2412. Accessed on 8 December 2025.

[12]'14 Causes of Upper Back Pain', *Florida Surgery Consultants*, 19 June 2020, https://tinyurl.com/bdza2um9. Accessed on 10 December 2025.

sensation is a cardiac emergency. Sometimes, the source is a strained muscle or an inflamed joint, not the heart's cry for help. Knowing the difference is crucial.

Cardiac Chest Pain: This pain is rarely sharp or fleeting. It is more often described as crushing, tight, heavy or suffocating (a force that seems to press inward rather than pierce). Many compare it to a weight on the chest, akin to having an elephant perched squarely over the sternum. This pain often radiates and may extend into various areas. It typically does not improve with posture changes or rest, and it is frequently accompanied by other symptoms.

Musculoskeletal Chest Pain: This pain, in contrast, tends to be sharper, more localized and clearly linked to movement or physical pressure. It may worsen when taking a deep breath, twisting the torso or pressing on the affected area. Common causes include overexertion, poor posture or minor trauma such as lifting something awkwardly or sleeping in an uncomfortable position. It is usually temporary and responds well to rest, gentle movement and mild pain relief.

Feature	*Cardiac Chest Pain*	*Musculoskeletal Chest Pain*
Nature of pain	Crushing, tight, heavy or squeezing	Sharp, stabbing or aching
Location	Centre or left side of chest	Localized to a specific area of the chest wall
Radiation	May spread to the jaw, neck, left arm, back or upper abdomen	Typically, does not radiate

Feature	*Cardiac Chest Pain*	*Musculoskeletal Chest Pain*
Trigger	Often occurs during exertion or stress	Triggered by movement, poor posture or physical activity
Relief	Not relieved by rest or change in posture	Worsens or improves with movement or pressing the area
Associated symptoms	Breathlessness, nausea, dizziness, cold sweats and fatigue	Usually isolated; may be tender to touch
Onset	Gradual or sudden, but persistent	Can be sudden and sharp, often linked to a specific action
Risk groups	More common and atypical in women, the elderly and diabetics	Common in athletes, in physically active individuals or after strain
Urgency	Medical emergency; requires immediate attention	Usually self-limiting; improves with rest or therapy

During a heart attack, people often react in two common but risky ways. Either they dismiss the pain, hoping it will pass, or they delay seeking help out of fear, confusion or denial. The correct response is immediate action. Call emergency services without delay, remain calm, sit or lie down and avoid exertion.

Nevertheless, the human body doesn't always follow textbook patterns when it comes to signalling distress, especially in women, older adults and those with diabetes. In such individuals, heart-related issues may present in less obvious ways than the classic chest pain. Instead, signs might include:

- Unexplained fatigue
- Mild discomfort in the back, shoulders or neck
- A sensation of indigestion or heartburn
- Anxiety or a sense of unease
- Shortness of breath without any chest discomfort

While these symptoms may often have harmless explanations, it is wise to stay attentive, particularly when they appear suddenly or feel out of character. Listening to your body is an act of self-respect. Think of it as responding to a subtle knock rather than waiting for a loud alarm.

The Lung Signals You Shouldn't Shrug Off

We often think of the heart as the central force driving life, beating rhythmically to sustain us. However, the lungs, often overlooked, are just as essential. The heart and lungs are close partners, where each breath we take is supported by the heart and where every beat relies on the oxygen the lungs deliver. When one falters, the other often follows, which is why issues with one can quickly affect the other.

Breathing difficulties, when ignored, can evolve from manageable to life-threatening. Here are some signs that may indicate a deeper problem:

- A sudden increase in fatigue, feeling winded after minimal exertion, like walking upstairs or carrying groceries

- Tightness in the chest that seems to worsen when in enclosed spaces or when you try to take a deep breath
- Difficulty lying flat at night as you struggle to find a position where you can breathe more easily
- An unusual wheeze when exhaling or a persistent cough that refuses to go away even after weeks
- A dull ache or discomfort across the upper back, often indicating a respiratory or circulatory issue

These subtle symptoms in the lungs are the body's early way of asking for attention. Persistent shortness of breath, wheezing or a lingering cough may signal chronic conditions like asthma, chronic obstructive pulmonary disease (COPD) or even heart failure.

Among the more urgent concerns is pulmonary embolism (PE), which is a condition where a blood clot blocks blood flow in the lungs. Though rare, it can develop suddenly and requires immediate medical care. Watch for symptoms such as:

- Sharp chest pain that worsens with deep breathing
- Sudden, unexplained breathlessness
- A rapid heart rate and dizziness or light-headedness
- In severe cases, coughing up blood

Furthermore, struggling to breathe while lying flat might simply be due to a chilly room or nasal congestion. However, when this discomfort persists or feels unnatural, it is worth paying attention. One often-overlooked reason is fluid buildup in the lungs caused by heart failure. If the heart can't pump blood effectively, fluid may back up into the lungs, making it harder to breathe when reclining.

While not every case is serious, it is always wise to listen to your body.

Breathing may feel like an automatic process, but it is anything but ordinary. The lungs and heart work tirelessly, moment by moment, to keep us alive. Pay attention to the alarms they send. A shortness of breath or a racing heart could be your body's way of asking for help, and the sooner you respond, the better.

The Breast Alarm

Breast health is often seen as a topic reserved solely for women, but that's a misconception which can have serious consequences. Both men and women need to understand that breast tissue is not only found in women but is present in everyone. For both women and men, the breast tissue can reveal early signs of health issues, many of which can be detected through simple, regular examinations. When approached with awareness, breast self-exams become a vital tool for early detection, helping individuals tune in to their bodies in a proactive manner.

Breast tissue is a dynamic part of the body, sensitive to hormonal changes, lifestyle factors and even environmental conditions. Recognizing normal variations and identifying abnormal changes early can make all the difference. Monthly self-examinations should be conducted with care, as they provide essential information about the state of the tissue. Rather than viewing the breast as a mere aesthetic feature, consider it a sensitive area that can communicate important health signals if properly understood.

Feel a Lump? Pause, Breathe, Check

While lumps are often benign, especially if they fluctuate with the menstrual cycle, any new or persistent lump should be investigated. A lump could signal a benign condition like a cyst or fibrocystic changes or it could be a sign of something more serious. When in doubt, a professional evaluation is essential.

Shape-Shifting Isn't Always Magic

Asymmetry is common and usually not a cause for concern, but sudden changes in the size or shape of the breasts could indicate an underlying issue. Such changes might signal growth within the breast tissue or structural changes caused by factors like inflammation or tumours. In men, a condition known as gynaecomastia, which causes the enlargement of male breast tissue, is often benign but should still be evaluated to rule out any other health concerns.

What's Normal, What's Not

The skin of the breast is a sensitive indicator of health. Changes such as dimpling, puckering or redness, especially when the skin starts to resemble the texture of an orange peel (peau d'orange), can be caused by a variety of conditions. Sometimes, these signs may result from harmless inflammation, allergic reactions or infections. However, in other cases, they may point to more serious issues like lymphatic blockage or a tumour near the surface.

Whether minor or significant, such skin changes deserve attention and a medical opinion, regardless of your gender.

Nipple Changes Explained

Any unexpected changes in the nipple such as inversion, retraction and unexplained discharge (especially if bloody) deserve attention. While such signs can stem from benign causes like infections or ductal inflammation, they may also indicate more serious conditions, including malignancy. Persistent itching or irritation could point to inflammatory skin issues or infections. It's important not to panic, but it's important not to dismiss these signs either.

The Many Faces of Breast Pain

Breasts, whether in men or women, are sensitive, responsive tissues that can speak volumes about your overall health. Hormonal fluctuations, infections, inflammation and tumours can all manifest through changes in the breast. Early detection of these changes can lead to better outcomes, particularly in conditions like breast cancer, where survival rates are significantly higher when detected early.[13]

While breast pain is often benign and cyclical, persistent or localized pain that doesn't correlate with the menstrual cycle should raise concern. Constant pain in one breast, especially if it is isolated to a specific area, might point to an underlying issue, requiring further examination.

Regular self-exams, conducted with care and attentiveness, can help individuals become familiar with their baseline breast tissue and recognize deviations from the norm. Just as we monitor other aspects of our health, such as blood pressure

---

[13]Sathishkumar, Krishnan, Jayasankar Sankarapillai, Aleyamma Mathew, Rekha A. Nair, Nitin Gangane, Sushma Khuraijam, Debabrata Barmon, Shashank Pandya, Gautam Majumdar, Vinay Deshmane, Eric Zomawia, Tseten Wangyal Bhutia, Kaling Jerang, Preethi Sara George, Swapna Maliye, Rajesh Laishram, Gaurav Das, Anand Shah, Shiromani Debbarma, Shravani Koyande, Lalawmpuii Pachuau, Ashok Sherpa, Gegong Jongkey, Meesha Chaturvedi, Priyanka Das, Stephen Santhappan, and Prashant Mathur, 'Breast Cancer Survival in India across 11 Geographic Areas under the National Cancer Registry Programme', *Cancer*, Vol. 130, No. 1, 2024, pp. 1816–25, https://doi.org/10.1002/cncr.35188. Accessed on 8 December 2025.

and cholesterol, regular monitoring of breast health can be empowering.

The Upper Back Edition

While poor posture and muscular strain are common causes of upper back discomfort, there are many other factors at play. Understanding the full spectrum of potential causes is essential to differentiating between mere strain and something far more critical. Let's explore the various underlying conditions that might be at the root of upper back pain.

Cracking the Thoracic Code

The thoracic spine, located between the neck and lower back, plays a vital role in maintaining your body's structure. When the discs in this region become herniated or misaligned or when degenerative changes occur, the pain can be deep, radiating and often unbearable. This kind of pain typically intensifies with certain movements or postures, and it may be felt across the upper back. Since this part of the spine is less flexible than the neck or lower back, issues here can significantly affect mobility and comfort.

Coughing, Wheezing, Gasping?

Sometimes, pain between the shoulder blades can be linked to lung conditions. Pneumonia, pleurisy (inflammation of the pleura, which is the lining around the lungs) and even lung cancer can cause upper back pain, especially when the irritation spreads to the pleura. This type of discomfort can often be mistaken for a muscle-related issue. If upper back pain is accompanied by coughing, shortness of breath or chest discomfort, it's essential to seek medical attention promptly.

The Emotional Baggage Claim

The upper back often serves as a 'storage space' for tension. The trapezius muscle, which spans the upper back and shoulders, tightens in response to stress, anxiety and emotional strain. This muscle tightness is often triggered by daily stresses, whether it's an overwhelming workload, familial concerns or emotional challenges. When this tension persists, it can manifest as muscle knots, spasms or chronic discomfort, making it a critical point to monitor when stress levels rise.

Could It Be Your Heart? Here's What to Know

Upper back pain can, in some cases, be an indication of heart problems, as mentioned earlier. Particularly in women and those with diabetes, a heart attack may present with pain between the shoulder blades, sometimes without the typical chest pain that most people associate with a heart attack.

So, it's important to pay attention if you experience:

- Persistent pain that doesn't improve with rest or stretches
- Pain that worsens at night or disrupts your sleep
- Unexplained weight loss, fatigue or coughing
- Pain that feels different from your usual muscular discomfort or that radiates to other areas

These are not simply signs of poor posture or overexertion. They are body alarms. By addressing the underlying causes, whether they be spinal, respiratory or even cardiac, you can take steps to prevent complications and protect your long-term health.

Standing Tall in Poise, Power and Purpose

In this chapter, we have delved into the intricate relationship between the chest, upper back and overall well-being. We have seen how subtle shifts in posture or discomfort can signal larger issues.

Thus, a healthy chest and upper back aren't just about avoiding pain. Rather, they are essential to maintaining our strength, confidence and resilience. Just as the power pose aligns the body for success, a body that maintains its alignment in daily life fosters a sense of inner strength and clarity. When we care for these areas, we invest not just in our physical health but in our ability to face the world head-on with poise, power and purpose.

The Gut Instincts

The lion rules not by force alone. Long before danger shows itself, he feels the shift in the wind and the tension in the air. His roar can roll across five miles of savannah, but it is his instinct that truly holds his pride together.

'Trust your gut' is both advice and anatomy. The human gut houses over 100 million neurons,[14] forming its own neural network known as the enteric nervous system. This system, embedded in the walls of your digestive tract, can operate independently of the brain. It perceives, processes and reacts with remarkable speed and subtlety, long before you consciously register that anything is wrong.

Your abdomen is the command centre. The stomach, liver, pancreas, intestines and reproductive organs share space in a tightly coordinated chamber where digestion, detoxification, metabolism and reproduction unfold continuously. When something affects that balance, abdominal pain is often the first alarm (sharp, dull, cramping or constant).

The gut reads your life and responds in real time.

Gut instincts are real. And more often than not, they are right.

---

[14]Goyal, Raj K., and Ikuo Hirano, 'The Enteric Nervous System', *New England Journal of Medicine*, Vol. 334, No. 17, 1996, pp. 1106–15, https://doi.org/10.1056/NEJM199607183350323. Accessed on 8 December 2025.

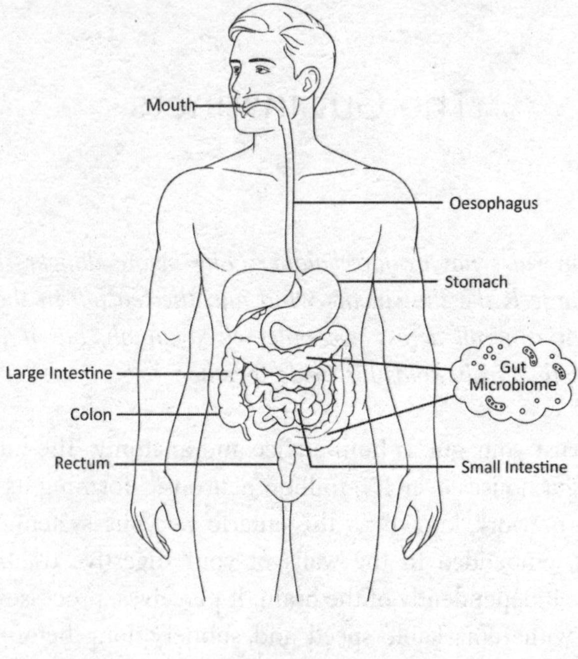

Figure 9: The gut

Your Abdomen Is Your Archive

We often refer to the region we call our 'stomach' as though it were a single organ, but in reality it's a much more complex system. It is where the liver defends, the pancreas calculates, the kidneys cleanse and the gut decides. It is also where cycles of menstruation churn, where trauma stores its secrets, where desire meets dysfunction and where disease whispers.

Children often clutch their stomachs when their hearts are afraid. We tend to dismiss it as 'tummy trouble' or 'just anxiety,' without realizing that the gut is the first place the body somatizes emotional pain. This is, therefore, not imagination but biology speaking through the bowels. And when we ignore that in children, we raise adults who apologize for their pain.

Women suffer quietly through endometriosis (a condition where the uterine lining grows where it's not supposed to), sometimes for years before being properly diagnosed. Men ignore gut pain, fearing weakness. Trauma survivors normalize the tightness that never leaves.

Yet, through it all, the abdomen continues to send vital alarms. Pay attention to it. It is your most honest plus-one.

Bloating and Belly Aches

Abdominal pain and bloating are among the most frequent complaints encountered in both clinics and households.

In its benign form, bloating may be nothing more than a post-lunch protest: too much food, too fast or too rich. Common causes include overeating, swallowing excess air (often unnoticed while talking and eating), food intolerances like lactose and gluten sensitivity, and transient gastrointestinal discomforts like irritable bowel syndrome (IBS). In such cases, symptoms often come and go, responding well to dietary changes, stress management and rest.

But then the belly has a darker side too. Certain gastrointestinal conditions, including some cancers like stomach, pancreatic and colorectal, can start quietly. Early signs might be subtle, such as mild abdominal pain, lingering bloating, changes in appetite or feeling full after just a few bites. These symptoms are easy to overlook or attribute to everyday habits but noticing them early can make all the difference.

Watch out for the following red flags:

- Persistent or worsening bloating that does not resolve with over-the-counter remedies

- Unexplained and unintentional weight loss
- A noticeable drop in appetite, or early satiety (feeling full quickly)
- A change in bowel habits lasting more than a few weeks
- Blood in the stool, even if occasional or minor
- A dull, nagging abdominal ache that's new and unexplained

Gut on Fire?

In some individuals, the issue may also stem from inflammatory conditions like Crohn's disease and ulcerative colitis, collectively known as inflammatory bowel disease (IBD). These are autoimmune conditions, meaning that the body's own defence system turns against it, leading to inflamed, ulcerated and damaged segments of the intestinal tract.

Symptoms here may not only include bloating and pain, but also:

- Chronic diarrhoea or constipation
- Fatigue
- Fever
- Unintended weight loss
- A persistent urge to empty the bowels without relief

Left untreated, these conditions can lead to serious complications, such as bowel strictures, fistulas or even cancer. Nevertheless, the good news is that, with modern medicine, they are manageable. The earlier these conditions are detected, the more effectively they can be controlled through medication, lifestyle changes or in some cases surgery.

Not Just in Your Gut, But in Your Mind Too

The gut is in constant conversation with the brain. There is an intimate, bidirectional relationship between mental health and gut health, often referred to as the gut-brain axis. Stress, anxiety and depression may very well exacerbate bloating and pain even in the absence of any physical disease. Functional disorders like IBS are perfect examples, wherein the symptoms are real and impactful but conventional tests often show little to no abnormality.

This doesn't mean the symptoms are 'all in your head.' Quite the opposite.

It's a vivid reminder that the body and mind are not separate entities and that they are woven from the same cloth.

The Shifting Tides of Digestion

When the System Speeds Up

Not all diarrhoea is dangerous (which is, basically, your body's way of quickly getting rid of something unwanted in your gut). A brief episode after a questionable meal or during a bout of flu is common. However, when diarrhoea overstays its welcome, persisting for more than a few days or returning regularly, it deserves your attention. The causes may range from gastrointestinal infections (viral, bacterial or parasitic) to malabsorption syndromes or chronic inflammatory conditions.

The warning signs intensify when diarrhoea is accompanied by:

- Blood or mucus in the stool
- High fever or significant fatigue
- Sudden weight loss
- Intense abdominal cramps

Notice the signs early before dehydration, weakness or strain set in. Acting sooner often leads to easier treatment and a quicker, smoother recovery.

When the System Slows Down to a Crawl

Equally important is the other extreme: constipation. It is defined not just by infrequent stools but also by difficulty, straining or the persistent feeling of incomplete evacuation. Chronic constipation may be a symptom of:

- Hypothyroidism, where metabolism slows across all systems
- Neurological conditions affecting gut motility
- Obstruction from benign polyps or dangerous masses
- Colorectal cancer, particularly in older adults or those with a family history

If you find yourself reaching for laxatives regularly, or feeling bloated, heavy and perpetually 'not quite done,' there might be a mechanical or functional problem in the pipeline.

This is especially critical when changes appear suddenly or dramatically, without any change in diet or routine.

The Gut's Scarlet Message

Among all bowel-related symptoms, the appearance of blood is the one that should never be ignored. Here's why:

Bright red blood	It usually comes from the lower gastrointestinal (GI) tract (closer to the exit). While often less serious, persistent bleeding should still be checked. Bright red blood may appear on the surface of the stool or on toilet paper.

Dark, tar-like stool	It indicates bleeding higher up in the digestive tract (stomach or small intestine). The dark, sticky look comes from digested blood and should be promptly checked by a doctor.
Intermittent or mixed bleeding	Bleeding may come and go or mix with stool, and it can occur anywhere along the colon. Early detection is important, so watch for changes in bowel habits, abdominal pain or unexplained weight loss.

Occasional spotting isn't always serious, but noticing patterns or changes early is helpful for overall digestive health.

Listen without Shame

There is a social silence around bowels. We are embarrassed to talk about our toilet habits, even to doctors. However, the truth is that your stool is a daily health report, which you should read, respect and report when needed.

Be proactive. Be specific.

When Weight Falls Away or Creeps Up

The body never changes its shape without a reason. Remember that.

Losing weight without trying may feel like a welcome surprise, but it can sometimes indicate that the body is working harder than usual. Conditions such as digestive disorders, thyroid imbalance or even chronic infections can affect how we absorb or use nutrients. In rare cases, it may signal something more serious, which is why noticing patterns early is so valuable.

On the other hand, unexplained weight gain isn't always about diet or lifestyle. Hormonal shifts, stress or certain medical conditions can play a part. Here, too, observing gradual changes and seeking guidance help ensure the body stays in balance.

The Takeaway

The body has a natural rhythm of fluctuation, but deviations beyond five per cent of your body weight in a few months, without conscious effort, should not be brushed off.

Think of unexplained weight change as a symptom, not as a standalone problem. A visible change often precedes an invisible one, sometimes hormonal, sometimes metabolic and sometimes more serious.

'I Want to Eat Your' Liver, Kidney, and Pancreas

The title evokes curiosity and, perhaps, discomfort. Inspired by the deeply reflective anime *I Want to Eat Your Pancreas*, this section aims to raise awareness about the liver, kidneys and pancreas—organs which are not celebrated in everyday conversation even though they are vital to life's internal equilibrium.

The liver metabolizes, synthesizes and neutralizes, processing everything from nutrients to medications. The kidneys calibrate fluid volume, filter waste and regulate electrolytes with mathematical precision. The pancreas releases enzymes and hormones which ensure that digestion and glucose balance remain stable.

These organs operate in concert, maintaining the body's inner order with a sophistication that is easy to overlook.

Yellow Isn't Always Sunshine

Jaundice is the yellowing of the skin and eyes. It's often the body's first visible alarm that the liver is under stress. While many think of hepatitis, jaundice can also reflect other liver concerns such as cirrhosis, bile duct blockage or, more rarely, cancer. It emerges when the liver struggles to process bilirubin (a natural by-product of red blood cell breakdown), causing it to build up and tint the skin and eyes.

Other liver clues may include fatigue, a sense of fullness or discomfort under the ribs on the right side, pale stools and dark urine. Seeking timely medical advice allows problems to be identified early, if any.

Puffs and Pulls

Swelling may arrive quietly, with just a subtle puffiness in the ankles at day's end, or with a waistline that feels tighter despite no change in diet. While it can result from a salty meal or long hours on your feet, persistent or unexplained swelling is the body's gentle signal to pay attention.

Oedema happens when fluid escapes the bloodstream and collects in tissues. Kidneys that aren't filtering efficiently or a heart that isn't pumping effectively, can allow fluid to build up in extremities, the abdomen or even the lungs. This can cause discomfort, affect movement and, in some cases, impact breathing or circulation. Although oedema can have benign causes, it may also indicate more serious conditions like kidney disease or heart failure.

Rapid swelling accompanied by fatigue, shortness of breath or general malaise deserves timely medical attention. Early awareness often helps prevent complications and allows for simpler, more effective interventions.

The Bitter Side of Sugar

Tucked behind the stomach, the pancreas governs blood sugar by releasing insulin, which is an indispensable hormone that helps cells absorb glucose for energy. When this finely tuned mechanism falters, sugar accumulates in the bloodstream, triggering the onset of diabetes. Symptoms of early diabetes often go unnoticed or are mistaken for everyday fatigue. These may include:

- Constant thirst that doesn't improve with fluid intake
- Frequent urination, especially at night
- Unexpected weight loss without changes in diet or activity
- Persistent tiredness, even after rest

Each of these signs reflects the body's increasing challenge in managing glucose. If left unchecked, the kidneys may gradually lose their ability to filter waste (a process known as diabetic nephropathy), often progressing silently until significant damage occurs, impacting nerves, eyes, blood vessels and the heart.

Recognizing these early signs and acting promptly can preserve organ function, keeping the body strong alongside the pancreas.

Menstrual Health, Shh...

The menstrual cycle is more than a calendar event. It is a finely tuned physiological process that shapes the well-being of countless bodies each month. However, despite its biological brilliance, it has long been shrouded in whispers, wrapped in myths and too often met with rolled eyes or nervous chuckles. From being labelled as impure to being wrongly seen as a monthly mood malfunction soothed only by chocolates, menstruation has been misunderstood for generations.

Behind the scenes, nevertheless, complex systems are at work. Each cycle, the body readies itself for the possibility of pregnancy by thickening the uterine lining, and it is an intricate process orchestrated by oestrogen and progesterone. If fertilization doesn't occur, the body sheds this lining in what is known as menstruation, which can slow digestion, alter bowel movements and trigger abdominal bloating, cramps or even urinary changes.

And herein lies the confusion: These signs often blur the line between what's considered 'normal' cycle-related discomfort and what could point to a deeper issue with conditions like endometriosis, fibroids and irritable bowel syndrome.

Dismissive attitudes don't help either.

Pain is waved off as exaggerated. Discomfort is branded as weakness. And ancient taboos still cast a shadow over open conversations, making it harder to recognize when something is amiss. It's time to move beyond outdated beliefs and hesitant silences.

Understanding how the menstrual cycle affects abdominal health is a human concern. Whether you experience these changes first-hand or care for someone who does, awareness bridges the gap between ignorance and intervention.

Period Pain Doesn't Have to Be Part of Life

Pain during menstruation is one of the most frequently reported forms of abdominal discomfort. Often described as a dull ache or sharp cramp in the lower abdomen, it can range from mildly annoying to completely incapacitating. The sensation stems from the uterus contracting to shed its lining.

- **Mild cramping** that begins just before or during menstruation is common and usually manageable with rest, hydration and over-the-counter pain relief.
- **Severe, throbbing or stabbing pain** that does not improve with medication or rest may indicate something serious.
- **Pain that radiates to the lower back or thighs** or continues well after the menstrual flow has ended, may be concerning.
- **Abdominal pain combined with unusually heavy bleeding**, clotting or fatigue could suggest an underlying gynaecological issue.
- **Persistent discomfort during intercourse, urination or bowel movements**, particularly around the menstrual cycle, is another concerning sign.

The key takeaway is simple: Regular, intense menstrual pain isn't something to be endured or joked about. Early diagnosis and management can make all the difference for long-term reproductive and general health.

The Monthly Swell

Abdominal bloating around the menstrual cycle often feels like an uninvited guest. Suddenly, everything feels tight, swollen and uncomfortable, as if the digestive system has gone on a protest. This sensation isn't imagined. It is a result of the body's natural hormonal fluctuations, particularly the rise in progesterone levels during the second half of the menstrual cycle.

Just track your symptoms and try gentle lifestyle adjustments. If discomfort persists or worsens, consult a healthcare professional for guidance.

Sexual Health Goes Beyond Sex

Sexual health is a crucial component of overall well-being, extending far beyond the act of intercourse. It encompasses the proper functioning of the reproductive organs, which are intricately linked to the abdomen and midsection. In both men and women, conditions affecting sexual health such as sexually transmitted infections (STIs), prostate issues, pelvic inflammatory disease (PID) and even issues like erectile dysfunction or uterine fibroids can manifest through abdominal pain, bloating and digestive discomfort.

In women, the uterus, ovaries and fallopian tubes are intimately connected with the gastrointestinal system. In men, the prostate, testicles and surrounding organs can also influence abdominal health. These organs impact each other in complex ways. For children and the elderly, sexual health issues may not be immediately obvious but still play a significant role in overall health. For example, young adolescents may experience abdominal discomfort linked to early sexual development or infections, while elderly individuals might face challenges like prostate enlargement or reduced hormonal levels that manifest as abdominal symptoms.

Modern lifestyles, with transient relationships and casual encounters, may heighten the risk of undiagnosed infections and sexual health complications. Unprotected encounters and neglecting regular check-ups can impact sexual health, leading to conditions that can affect fertility, cause chronic pain or even result in long-term complications.

From adolescents to the elderly, understanding and caring for sexual health is vital not just for intimacy but for a healthy life and overall well-being.

The Pelvic Problem No One Talks about

Pelvic inflammatory disease (PID) is an infection of the internal reproductive organs, most often triggered by untreated sexually transmitted infections like chlamydia or gonorrhoea. In women, it affects the uterus, fallopian tubes and ovaries. In men, though PID itself doesn't occur, they are often the asymptomatic carriers and transmitters of the infections that cause it. This makes men an inseparable part of both the problem and the solution.

PID creates ripple effects through families, partners, communities and generations, and it often starts with something subtle:

- A persistent ache in the lower abdomen or pelvis
- Pain during or after sexual activity
- Fever, fatigue or abnormal discharge
- Painful urination, irregular periods or nausea

For some, the pain is occasional. For others, it is a chronic torment that becomes a new normal. Too many don't even know it's happening until it's too late.

When the Infection Strikes Deep

PID can permanently harm reproductive organs, sometimes causing ectopic pregnancies where a fertilized egg implants outside the womb, often in a scarred fallopian tube (which is a life-threatening situation). Further, chronic pelvic pain may persist for years, affecting mental health, relationships and overall quality of life. In severe cases, the infection can spread into the bloodstream, causing sepsis (a dangerous systemic response where the body attacks its own organs and tissues).

And it's not only women who are affected. Men who

carry or transmit the STIs responsible for PID can experience testicular pain, prostatitis and long-term complications too. They are not immune. They are often just uninformed.

Why All This Still Happens

Because shame still overrides science. Because sex education is still broken, filtered through discomfort and denial. Because people assume they are 'clean' if they feel fine. Because routine STI screening isn't embedded into adult healthcare, especially for men. And because abdominal and pelvic pain is still often dismissed, especially in women and gender-diverse individuals, as 'just stress,' 'just periods' and 'nothing serious.'

What Needs to Change

Whether you are a teenager exploring intimacy, a man in a long-term relationship, a woman planning for a family or a senior navigating new chapters, you are not exempt from the consequences of hidden infections. Therefore, annual STI testing must become routine, not optional, regardless of symptoms, gender or relationship status. Pain must be investigated. STIs must lose the stigma.

Partners must be part of the process. If one is diagnosed, both need treatment. Otherwise, it is a revolving door of reinfection.

Winning Life, Slumdog Millionaire-Style

Listening closely is your gut instinct, your internal Jamal, noticing what others overlook. Track patterns, respond early, nourish your core and seek guidance when something feels off. Every alarm guides you towards balance, resilience and strength. Your gut senses first, acts first and remembers every detail. Heed it, and you turn whispers into advantage, discomfort into insight and the wisdom of your abdomen into a winning strategy for life.

The Lesson in Charlie Chaplin's Gait

Charlie Chaplin's shuffle was a masterclass in the art of movement. His turned-out feet, knocking knees and awkward steps told a story of vulnerability that captivated millions. But what did it really say about him?

Chaplin's genius lay in turning imperfection into brilliance, reminding us that how we move speaks volumes about our bodies and our lives. Michael Jackson also didn't just walk. He glided. His moonwalk, liquid and effortless, revealed a different kind of mastery. Also, Mr Bean, bumbling and unpredictable, made every misstep charming.

These 'quirky' gaits embodied control, balance and presence. They showed us how much power lies in the way we move.

However, while these performances were a celebration of movement's potential, they also serve as an alarm for us. These iconic figures, in their genius, remind us of the delicate balance we often take for granted. What if our own bodies aren't performing at their best? What if, like Chaplin's shuffle, our body is silently struggling beneath the surface?

Trust me, you don't want to be left hobbling without a backup plan. And the best part? You don't have to hobble at all if you start paying attention now.

If Movement Had an Engine, This Would Be It

The lower back (also known as the lumbar spine) and hips are the engine room of movement, quietly carrying the weight of everything we do.

The lumbar spine, which is made of five strong vertebrae with soft, flexible discs between them, provides both stability and mobility while protecting the nerves that send signals between the brain and body. The hips are ball-and-socket joints where the thigh bone meets the pelvis. Their design lets us bend, twist, walk and run, while cartilage cushions the joints and absorbs impact. When these areas are strained, worn or injured, movement can feel stiff, awkward or painful. That is why understanding how they work is so important.

Working together, the lower back and hips create the foundation for posture, balance and every step we take.

A Pain in the 'Back-End'

Did you know that lower back pain is the leading cause of disability worldwide? According to the World Health Organization (WHO), more than 600 million people live with it daily.[15] It is so common that it is often mistaken for normal. However, persistent lower back pain can serve as an important alarm from your body, highlighting issues that may need attention.

Sometimes, it points to kidney problems that need care. Sometimes, it signals spinal nerves under pressure. And sometimes, it indicates irritation of the sciatic nerve, affecting daily movement. Paying attention to these signs can help you address problems early.

---

[15]World Health Organization, 'Low Back Pain', *World Health Organization*, 19 June 2023, https://tinyurl.com/akz68bde. Accessed on 8 December 2025.

That One-Sided Ache Could Be Your Kidneys Talking

That deep, one-sided ache in your lower back might feel like a pulled muscle, but if it lingers despite rest and painkillers, it may not be musculoskeletal at all. It could be your kidneys. Kidney infections and stones often present as a dull, cramping pain just below the ribcage, which doesn't improve with stretching, heat or massage.

Muscle pain usually responds to rest. Kidney-related pain doesn't.

Imagine a machine working nonstop and filtering around 50 gallons of fluid every single day. That's your kidneys. They regulate blood pressure, flush out waste and keep your body in balance.

Even a tiny hiccup in kidney function can ripple across your system, affecting energy, focus and overall health.

So, look out for:

- Persistent one-sided lower back ache
- Fever and chills
- Nausea and vomiting
- Cloudy, foul-smelling or bloody urine
- Pain or burning sensation while urinating
- Frequent or urgent need to urinate

If you notice these symptoms, don't wait. See a doctor.

Painkillers may relieve discomfort, but only tests like a urine analysis, blood work or an ultrasound can reveal the underlying cause and help you take the right steps to protect your health.

The Stiff Pull after Carrying Groceries Upstairs

Carrying heavy groceries upstairs can sometimes trigger a subtle stiffness in your lower back.

Your spine is a structural wonder: 24 vertebrae stacked with precision, cushioned by fluid-filled discs and laced with nerves that relay signals faster than any broadband connection. However, when even one disc slips, dries out or collapses, the pain can be profound. Conditions like herniated discs, spinal stenosis and degenerative disc disease often begin with a stiffness here, a twinge there or a subtle ache that lingers after bending or lifting.

Addressing the alarms early allows you to take steps like gentle stretching, proper posture or medical guidance to protect your spine.

Watch for:

- Stiffness or sharp pain during bending or twisting
- Pain that worsens with prolonged sitting or standing
- Tingling or numbness in the buttocks, legs or feet
- Weakness in one leg or dragging of the foot
- Discomfort that radiates downward with movement

Creaks, Clicks and Persistent Stiffness

Osteoarthritis is one of the leading causes of hip pain, particularly in older adults. As the cartilage that cushions the hip joint deteriorates, the bones begin to rub against each other, causing pain, stiffness and inflammation. This degenerative process can gradually limit the range of motion, making it difficult to perform even simple tasks such as walking, climbing stairs and sitting for prolonged periods. In fact, by age 60, nearly 25 per cent of people will exhibit signs of hip arthritis on X-rays, though symptoms may not always be present.[16]

While high-impact activities can sometimes aggravate joints, low-impact, weight-bearing exercises such as Tai Chi can be particularly beneficial. This gentle form of exercise helps improve joint flexibility, balance and strength without putting too much strain on the hip joint. Research has shown that Tai Chi can reduce pain and improve joint function in people with osteoarthritis, particularly in the knees and hips.[17]

There is a range of other strategies as well, from targeted physiotherapy to smart lifestyle adjustments, which can help preserve joint health. With mindful attention and timely care, the hips can remain resilient partners in movement well into later life.

Your Legs Up Close

Let's start with a chilling image: With every step you take, your knees absorb a force equivalent to three to five times your body weight.

It means that if you weigh 70 kilograms, each knee is taking around 350 kilograms of pressure with each stride. Now, picture yourself running. That force surges up to 1,000 kilograms per knee. Your knees and supporting structures are

---

[16]Singh, Ambrish, et al., 'Burden of Osteoarthritis in India and its States, 1990–2019: Findings from the Global Burden of Disease Study 2019', *Osteoarthritis and Cartilage*, Vol. 30, No. 8, 2022, pp. 1070–78, https://doi.org/10.1016/j.joca.2022.05.004. Accessed on 8 December 2025.

[17]Fransen, Marlene, Lillias Nairn, Julie Winstanley, Paul Lam, and John Edmonds, 'Physical Activity for Osteoarthritis Management: A Randomized Controlled Clinical Trial Evaluating Hydrotherapy or Tai Chi Classes', *Arthritis & Rheumatism*, Vol. 57, No. 3, 2007, pp. 407–14, https://doi.org/10.1002/art.22621. Accessed on 8 December 2025.

remarkably strong, specifically built to handle these loads.

The femur (your thigh bone) channels weight downward to the tibia, with the knee acting as a hinge stabilized by ligaments and cartilage. The anterior cruciate ligament (ACL) controls forward motion, while the menisci cushion impact and stabilize the joint. Unlike bones, cartilage doesn't heal easily, and damage over time can lead to osteoarthritis. Lower down, the calves act as muscular pumps, helping blood return to the heart, while the Achilles tendon, the strongest tendon in the body, connects calf muscles to the heel and enables powerful movement.

Healthy muscles, ligaments and alignment keep your legs resilient, supporting every step, jump and run.

When Your Leg's Traffic Jam Slows You Down

Blood must defy gravity every second to return from your feet to your heart. When that system weakens, the fluid pools and the pressure builds.

Swelling that lingers, especially in the lower legs or ankles, could be the body's way of saying, 'I'm struggling.' It often occurs when the valves in your veins aren't working optimally, causing blood to pool instead of flowing smoothly back to the heart. Recognizing this early gives you the chance to take steps like movement, gentle exercises or professional guidance.

Varicose veins (that is, swollen, twisted veins that press against the skin like blue ropes) may be the next chapter. They often arrive with an ache, a heaviness or the sense that your legs are carrying more than their share.

And when discolouration, warmth or tenderness strikes one leg more than the other, the stakes rise sharply. These could be early indicators of deep vein thrombosis (that is, a clot hidden deep in the venous system). If ignored, it can break loose, travel to the lungs and cause serious complications.

When Leg Nerves Start Sending Mixed Signals

The nervous system flickers, and in the legs, those flickers matter. Your legs and feet may begin to feel strange with these symptoms:

- Numbness that creeps in without warning
- Tingling like insects crawling beneath the skin
- Burning that intensifies at night
- Sudden weakness or a sense of instability
- Sharp, electric pains that shoot unpredictably
- A loss of the ability to feel temperature or texture

These symptoms can be early signs of peripheral neuropathy (a condition in which nerves gradually lose function). It can result from diabetes, nutritional gaps or reduced circulation.

Identifying the cause early allows for interventions, such as better blood sugar management, nutritional support or improved circulation.

Knee-d for Caution

Knees are intricate joints under constant stress. Sudden twists, falls or impacts can injure ligaments or the meniscus, producing pain, swelling or instability. Other changes like morning stiffness, occasional swelling or subtle locking may indicate early joint degeneration. At this stage, targeted exercises, controlled movement and maintaining a healthy load on the joint can help preserve function. Persistent pain or instability warrants assessment, as early insight often determines long-term knee health.

Feet in Focus

Take a moment now. Sit down. Look at your feet. Not just glance but really see them. How do they rest on the floor? Are your toes curled, flattened or turned outward? Do the bones protrude oddly? Though feet and ankles are the furthest points from the heart and brain, every contour of the foot tells a story of your gait, your habits and your health.

Bunions, hammer toes and collapsed arches often reflect compensations made silently over the years while standing unevenly, walking imprecisely and overloading joints above.

Flat feet may cause misalignments all the way up to the neck. A fallen arch may rotate the knees inward, twist the hips or throw the spine off-centre without any conscious awareness.

Cold, numb or tingling feet may signal compromised blood flow or nerve function (symptoms also common in diabetes, peripheral artery disease or neuropathy). If your feet seem oddly pale, purple or 'asleep,' more often than not something may be misfiring in your circulatory or nervous systems.

Feet can change subtly over time, often without pain, and maintaining their resilience is key to long-term comfort and mobility.

Footwear plays a major role in this. Shoes that support natural alignment, allow proper circulation and protect your feet help preserve their strength and function.

Micro-Movers, Maximum Impact

Ankles are micro-adjusters, constantly recalibrating with each step to keep you upright. They handle thousands of directional shifts each day, and one missed cue has the power to undo years of balance.

Swelling around the ankle joint may seem like fluid retention or fatigue, but it may also indicate that veins, joints or the lymphatic system are under extra stress. Noticing this early allows you to support these systems through movement, circulation-friendly practices and professional guidance.

Stiffness or reduced mobility, especially after periods of rest, might be your first encounter with chronic inflammation.

Painful flare-ups, even without clear injury, could signal microfractures from repetitive stress or gout (a buildup of uric acid crystals often misread as a twisted ankle or sprain).

Watch how your ankles move when you walk. Do they seem rigid or overly flexible? This reflects your posture in motion; and how well your ankles function determines how well you move through space.

So, look again. Trace the bones with your fingers. Press the arch. Rotate your ankle. Notice the small pains and the silent compensations.

A Self-Check Table for Feet and Ankles

Check Area	*What to Observe*	*What It Could Mean*
Colour and temperature	Pale, bluish, blotchy skin; feet colder than hands	Your blood may not be circulating efficiently, which can happen if veins are struggling or circulation is slowed
Sensation	Numbness, tingling, dullness or 'dead spots' in toes and soles	Nerves in your feet may be under stress, sometimes due to early nerve changes or conditions like diabetes

Check Area	*What to Observe*	*What It Could Mean*
Pressure and pain	Tenderness in heel, ball or sides of feet; deep and lingering aches	Could indicate extra strain on joints, muscles, or soft tissues from overuse or early wear
Nails and skin	Thickened, discoloured nails; dry, cracked or unusually thin skin	May reflect minor infections, reduced circulation or nutrient gaps
Mobility and balance	Wobbling ankles, trouble rising on toes and poor balance on one foot	Shows that joints and muscles might be weakening slightly, affecting stability and coordination

The Torso-Limb Connection

In Kathak, a seasoned dancer can execute around a hundred footwork strikes per minute, each one precise, thunderous and rhythmically aligned with complex 'taals'.

The torso, your body's central pillar, is far more than a passive structure holding organs in place. It is the site of constant micro-adjustments, muscle firings and spinal negotiations that let you stand upright, bend, twist or even breathe with ease. It anchors and communicates with your lower extremities through a sophisticated network of muscles, fascia, joints and nerves, relaying cues and absorbing shocks in real time. Your legs, on the other hand, are not mere tools of locomotion. They are weight-bearers, stabilizers and levers of kinetic force. They allow for grace under pressure, whether in a ballet pirouette or a stumble averted on a wet floor.

This chapter explored the silent alliance between your torso and lower limbs and how they operate in synergy. When this relationship is intact, movement feels fluid, balanced and effortless. However, when something disrupts it, such as a weak core, a stiff hip or a neglected ankle, the consequences ripple upward and downward in a kinetic chain reaction. A knee pain may originate in your spine, and a back ache might be birthed in your hamstrings.

So, the next time you sit with ease or rise without groaning, pause. Your torso and lower limbs have struck another perfect accord.

More Than Skin, Hair and Nails

Frida Kahlo's bold, unapologetic appearance wasn't just a style statement. Her unibrow, moustache and traditional Mexican attire became acts of resistance that confronted beauty standards.

The human body is an intricate record of time. From the first wrinkle to the last strand of hair, every change carries a story. Beyond the obvious wrinkles and greying hair, the real science of ageing is itself embedded in the very fibres of our skin, hair and nails. These seemingly mundane features offer a wealth of information about our chronological and biological age, and forensic scientists have learned to figure out these secrets with remarkable precision.

For example, forensic experts can determine age by analysing the elasticity of the skin (a process that directly correlates with the breakdown of collagen over time). As we age, the collagen fibres in our skin become more rigid and less organized, causing the skin to lose its elasticity. The presence of fine lines, particularly around the eyes, is one of the clearest indicators of this process, and experts can determine a person's age by studying the depth and number of these lines.

Similarly, the condition of hair can provide a forensic timeline. Hair growth cycles as well as the rate of hair loss are influenced by a complex interplay of hormones, diet and stress. For instance, younger individuals generally have a higher percentage of growing (anagen) hair, while older individuals may experience a shift towards more dormant hair follicles (telogen).

Perhaps the most surprising truth lies in your nails. The shape, colour or texture of your nails can reveal crucial insights into your heart health, liver function or even hidden infections. In fact, nails are so precise in their forensic value that pathologists often turn to them first in unexplained cases.

If the Skin Could Talk...

When we think about our skin, the first image that comes to mind is usually the face. We wash it with face wash, pamper it with face packs and carefully apply moisturizers. However, the health of our skin extends far beyond just the face, covering every inch of our body, from the delicate skin of our private parts to the often-neglected underarms.

The skin consists of three primary layers, namely the epidermis, dermis and hypodermis. The epidermis acts as the outermost layer, providing a barrier against the elements, while the dermis is where most of the skin's essential functions occur, such as temperature regulation, sensation and the production of collagen and elastin. Beneath this lies the hypodermis, or subcutaneous layer, which stores fat and helps insulate the body. When any of these layers is affected, the skin gives clues.

Freckles, Spots and Fascination

Freckles and age spots have long been symbols of sun-kissed beauty, but are they just harmless remnants of time spent in the sun, or do they hold deeper insights into your health? In many cultures, freckles are seen as charming or even considered marks of youth and vitality. In fact, people with lighter skin of certain descent are more prone to develop freckles due to genetic predisposition.[18] However, these seemingly innocent spots (small, brownish marks that appear on the face, shoulders or arms) may signal much more than just a history of UV exposure in some cases.

It's, therefore, not the existence of these marks that should raise concern but rather their sudden changes. If a freckle or sunspot begins to grow larger, change in colour or develop uneven edges, it may indicate a need for medical attention as it could occasionally signal skin conditions such as melanoma. Men over 50 are slightly more at risk, so being attentive to the skin is a helpful and proactive habit.

In many cultures, the changing hues of a woman's skin during pregnancy or as a result of birth control use are considered part of the natural ageing process. Some of these changes, however, may reflect internal hormonal shifts. Melasma, often referred to as the 'mask of pregnancy,' manifests as dark, irregular patches, typically on the forehead, cheeks or upper lip. This condition occurs when hormonal fluctuations, particularly elevated oestrogen and progesterone levels, trigger excess melanin production. While more common among women of Latin, Asian or Middle Eastern descent, it affects women worldwide.

It's essential to remember that melasma isn't limited to pregnancy or hormonal changes. It can also result from

---

[18]Yamaguchi, Kyoko, Chiaki Watanabe, Akira Kawaguchi, Takehiro Sato, Izumi Naka, Misaki Shindo, Keiichi Moromizato, Kenichi Aoki, Hajime Ishida, and Ryosuke Kimura, 'Association of Melanocortin 1 Receptor Gene (MC1R) Polymorphisms with Skin Reflectance and Freckles in Japanese,' *Journal of Human Genetics*, Vol. 57, No. 11, 2012, pp. 700–08, https://doi.org/10.1038/jhg.2012.96. Accessed on 8 December 2025.

prolonged sun exposure, making sunscreen use even more critical in managing skin health.

Cultural Perception of Pigmentation

Around the globe, skin pigmentation and its variations are seen through different cultural lenses. In Western cultures, fair skin has often been idealized while darker skin tones have historically been subject to prejudice. This has led to an industry of skin-lightening products in places like South Asia where lighter skin is still sometimes equated with higher social status or beauty. In contrast, other parts of the world embrace darker skin tones as symbols of beauty and strength.

Regardless of how we culturally perceive these changes, they are biologically tied to how the body reacts to environmental, hormonal and lifestyle changes.

So, the next time you notice a freckle that wasn't there before or a patch of skin that has suddenly darkened, take a moment to understand its story. Your skin is a powerful, living map of your health, constantly updating itself with each passing day. Whether you are male or female, just pay attention.

Skin That Lives in the Shadows

Most skincare routines stop at the jawline or, at best, the elbows. However, the skin under your arms, between your legs and beneath your socks isn't just along for the ride. If you are not listening, you are missing some of the body's earliest alarms.

Underarms

Think your underarms are just about body odour? Not quite. These small, often-shaved patches of skin are surprisingly diagnostic. Darkening here isn't always from friction, razors or harsh deodorants. One common reason is acanthosis nigricans (AN) (a condition marked by velvety, hyperpigmented patches). While often mistaken for cosmetic discolouration, it may be an early indicator of insulin resistance, polycystic ovary syndrome (PCOS) or thyroid dysfunction.

This area is also a hotspot for contact dermatitis due to the high use of fragranced products, antiperspirants and shaving creams. The skin here is thinner and more permeable, making it vulnerable to irritation or inflammation. Infections like intertrigo (a rash caused by friction and trapped moisture) can also develop in the warm, enclosed environment of the underarm.

Therefore, unexplained dark patches, skin tags or persistent irritation should not be dismissed as hygiene issues. If discolouration persists despite exfoliation or skincare, skip the whitening creams. Ask for blood work to rule out the respective issues.

'Private Parts'

The skin in your genital area is the most absorbent, most reactive and often the most overlooked. Persistent itching, rashes, bumps or discolouration may sometimes signal a range of underlying concerns, from hormonal fluctuations or fungal overgrowth to sexually transmitted infections (STIs) or chronic conditions like lichen sclerosus (LS), which is often misdiagnosed as a simple yeast infection.

Because this skin is thinner and more permeable than elsewhere on the body, it is also more susceptible to irritants. Harsh soaps, synthetic underwear or tight clothing can trap moisture and cause friction, leading to bacterial or fungal flare-ups. Fragranced vaginal washes and douches may promise 'freshness' but often disrupt the natural microbiome, leaving the skin more vulnerable.

Many skin issues in these areas are benign and easily treatable. Nonetheless, even subtle changes, such as dryness, persistent redness or recurring inflammation, deserve attention. In men, irritation in the groin or scrotal area may reflect fungal infections or contact dermatitis, often dismissed out of embarrassment.

Feet

Your feet handle the weight of your day quite literally. Still, most people don't inspect them until there is pain. Cracked heels? May indicate vitamin deficiencies or dehydration. Unusual dryness or thickening? May signal circulatory issues or fungal infections like tinea pedis (athlete's foot).

Interesting fact: Foot odour isn't just about sweat. Rather, it's about bacteria digesting the sweat. More bacteria means a stronger smell. And if one foot smells worse than the other, you might be favouring that leg unconsciously, possibly due to a postural imbalance.

So, rotate your shoes. Wash feet with an antimicrobial soap, dry thoroughly, especially between the toes, and moisturize daily. Avoid lotion between the toes to prevent fungal overgrowth.

Nutritional Deficiencies

Dry, flaky or lacklustre skin may signal internal nutritional gaps. Deficiencies in vitamins A, C, D, E and the B-complex group don't just dull your glow but they also compromise the skin's structural integrity and ability to repair itself.

Vitamin A is essential for skin cell turnover. A lack of it may lead to rough, bumpy textures.

Vitamin C is a collagen co-factor, and its deficiency weakens skin elasticity and delays healing.

Vitamin D (synthesized through sun exposure) plays a key role in skin immunity and inflammation control.

Vitamin E (a powerful antioxidant) protects against oxidative stress from pollution and UV rays.

B-complex vitamins (especially B3 and B7) are vital for hydration, oil regulation and maintaining a healthy skin barrier.

Even the skin of sensitive regions such as underarms, feet and genital areas could reflect these deficiencies through unusual dryness, irritation or slow healing after minor trauma.

Tip: A nutrient-rich diet with leafy greens, nuts, seeds, fatty fish, citrus fruits and whole grains can dramatically improve overall skin resilience. Don't underestimate hydration either. Water is a nutrient too.

Your Hair Speaks Volumes

Hair doesn't grow or fall without reason. Each strand begins in a follicle anchored in the dermis, fed by capillaries, governed by hormones and influenced by stress, diet or disease.

The Thinning Tale

Sudden hair fall sometimes reflects underlying disorders, such as thyroid dysfunction, iron-deficiency anaemia, PCOS and even autoimmune conditions like alopecia areata. Emotional trauma may also shock the follicles into dormancy (telogen effluvium), causing widespread loss weeks after the trigger.

The Science beneath the Texture, Strength and Shine

Dry, brittle, or dull hair typically signals protein, vitamin B12, vitamin D, zinc or iron deficiencies. Even over-shampooing, especially with harsh sulphates, may sometimes strip the scalp's protective oils and disrupt its microbiome.

Body Hair Growth

Hair is hormonally driven. That's why androgens (like testosterone and DHT) govern not only scalp hair loss but also body hair growth.

Observation	*Possible Interpretation*	*Level of Urgency*
Thick hair on arms, back or chest (in women)	May suggest androgen excess (for example, PCOS and adrenal disorders)	Requires a hormonal evaluation
Sparse body hair (in men)	Could indicate testosterone deficiency or pituitary dysfunction	Warrants an endocrine review
Localized hair loss	Often due to fungal infections or autoimmune conditions (for example, alopecia areata)	Dermatological assessment is advised
Changes in colour or growth rate	Linked to ageing, chronic stress or medication side effects	No immediate intervention is needed if the condition remains stable

Don't ignore sudden body hair changes. Chart them, track patterns and test hormones.

Rotate shampoos if you use styling products as the residue may mimic scalp disorders. To prevent hair removal irritation or infections, use clean tools, avoid shared razors and always moisturize post-shave.

Nails Speak in Hues

The shape, colour and growth patterns of nails also reflect subtle nutrient imbalances to chronic disease indicators when interpreted carefully.

Nail Colour	*Possible Interpretation*	*Level of Urgency*
Bluish or purplish tint	Indicates reduced oxygen supply; may be linked to lung or cardiovascular conditions	Needs evaluation, especially if paired with breathlessness
Yellowing	Common in fungal infections; also seen in diabetes or thyroid issues	Observe its persistence
White or pale nails	May reflect anaemia, liver dysfunction or low protein levels	Investigate if accompanied by fatigue or poor appetite
Dark vertical streak	Can be benign (especially in darker skin); rarely indicates subungual melanoma	See a dermatologist if it changes in width or colour
Green or brownish hue	Often caused by bacterial infection (for example, pseudomonas) or trauma	Treat promptly if odour or swelling is present

Routine changes may mean nothing but persistent, unexplained alterations require closer scrutiny.

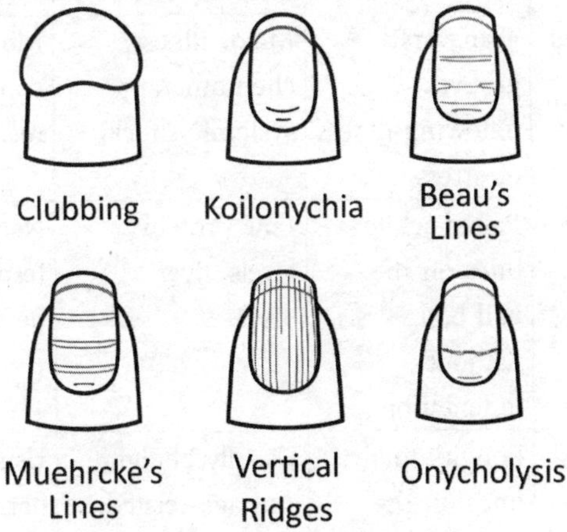

Figure 10: Shape and texture abnormalities in nails

Shape and Texture Abnormalities

Feature	*Description*	*What It May Sometimes Indicate*	*Urgency*
Clubbing	Nails curve around enlarged fingertips	Chronic lung disease, congenital heart disorders	Seek medical evaluation soon
Koilonychia	Spoon-shaped, concave nails	Iron-deficiency anaemia	Worth investigating

Feature	*Description*	*What It May Sometimes Indicate*	*Urgency*
Beau's lines	Transverse grooves following illness or stress	Major illness, chemotherapy, systemic shock	Monitor and consult if recurring
Muehrcke's lines	Paired white lines on the nail bed, without indentation	Low protein levels, liver disease	Needs lab testing if persistent
Vertical ridges	Longitudinal lines on the nail surface	Usually benign and age-related; malnutrition if severe	Usually harmless; monitor
Onycholysis	Nail lifting from the nail bed	Hyperthyroidism, fungal infections, or drug side effects	Investigate if widespread or persistent

Understanding Nail Patterns as Health Indicators

If you have been dealing with persistent fungal infections in your toenails, especially if you are older, diabetic, an athlete or have circulation issues, it's important to look beyond the surface. Recurring or treatment-resistant nail infections may sometimes reflect underlying problems in your immune function, vascular health or metabolic balance.

Alternatively, if you have noticed that they are growing more slowly, becoming thinner or changing shape without a clear external cause, it may be a sign of hypothyroidism, poor circulation or nutritional deficiencies that interrupt keratin production.

Some nail changes are harmless and age-related. But if you see ongoing discolouration, detachment or distortion, especially alongside fatigue, unexpected weight changes or shortness of breath, don't ignore it. Listen early and act decisively.

I Know What You Are Thinking…

It is easy to feel like everything is a symptom; every dry patch, every hair fall, every brittle nail. However, you scroll through hundreds of brands, opinions or ads each day without hesitation. Just imagine if you gave even a sliver of that attention to your own body. It doesn't even require a medical degree.

Also, think back to a time when women who knew how to read the body (for example, herbalists, midwives and early healers) were branded as witches. Why? Because they paid attention and they noticed when skin turned sallow, when hair thinned in grief or when nails lost their shine. In a world that feared what it didn't understand, awareness was power.

You don't need to be mystical to reclaim that power.

You just need to be curious and attentive.

The Young, the Old and the Language of the Body

A fading photograph holds details you didn't notice at first, such as a hand half-cut, a shadow too long or a smile that didn't reach the eyes. The photograph tells a deeper story of someone missing, of a truth just out of frame and of time already slipping away.

A child once deemed lazy, disobedient and inattentive stood at the heart of the film *Taare Zameen Par*. His teachers saw a boy uninterested in learning; his parents, a problem to be fixed. This cinematic portrayal reflects a real-world phenomenon. In both the very young and the very old, the body speaks a language that often goes unnoticed or misinterpreted (which, in this case, was dyslexia).

Children and the elderly, though vastly different in biology and life stage, share this one critical trait that they both rely heavily on non-verbal cues to express distress. Their physiological and psychological alarms rarely follow textbook presentations. A child may show an ear infection not through complaint but by tugging at the ear and crying inconsolably. An elderly patient may not report chest pain during a heart attack but might suddenly appear confused or withdrawn. These deviations are patterned, predictable and rooted in developmental and degenerative processes.

Scientific literature affirms that the immature nervous system of a child and the ageing body of an elder often communicate distress through indirect signs.[19] In children, the myelination of nerves, still incomplete in early years, alters sensory perception and response. In elders, diminished pain sensitivity, altered thermoregulation and cognitive decline mask classical symptoms. This makes clinical vigilance and intuitive/informed caregiving vital.

Body Alarms in Children

Developmental Considerations

Understanding the developmental context is crucial in deciphering body alarms in children. Unlike adults, children are not fully equipped to identify, interpret or articulate internal discomfort or physiological changes. Their responses, often behavioural, subtle or paradoxical, are shaped by the maturation of their nervous, immune and endocrine systems.

Infants (0–12 months)

Infants are almost entirely non-verbal. Their primary communication is through reflexes, cries, body movements and facial expressions. Body alarms in this stage can be easy to miss because symptoms may present non-specifically.

---

[19]UNICEF, 'How to Recognize Signs of Distress in Children', *UNICEF* Parenting, https://tinyurl.com/3n2ehtw9. Accessed on 3 September 2025; 'Ageing Changes in the Nervous System', *MedlinePlus Medical Encyclopaedia*, 15 July 2024, https://tinyurl.com/2v3sjj22. Accessed on 8 December 2025.

Normal Responses	*Concerning Signs*
Crying during hunger, overstimulation or discomfort	Persistent high-pitched or weak cry and extreme irritability
Sneezing, hiccups or mild temperature instability	Bulging fontanelle, poor feeding and reduced urine output
Startle reflex (Moro), rooting and grasping are normal primitive reflexes	Grunting, nasal flaring or chest retractions (signs of respiratory distress)

While the concerning signs sometimes indicate serious conditions such as meningitis, sepsis or congenital heart disease, they also often reflect normal variations in infant behaviour.

Prompt evaluation helps ensure infants stay healthy and receive timely care when needed.

Toddlers (1–3 years)

Toddlers are at the cusp of developing speech but rely heavily on gestures and behaviour to express illness. Their immune systems are still maturing and symptoms may be masked by emotional volatility.

Normal Responses	*Concerning Signs*
Short attention spans and emotional outbursts	Inconsolable crying or sudden silence (or refusal to bear weight or walk)
Mild fevers with viral illnesses	Persistent vomiting or dehydration signs (for example, sunken eyes and dry mouth)

Normal Responses	*Concerning Signs*
Night waking, picky eating and mild regression during stress	Sudden changes in behaviour (aggression, apathy or fearfulness)

Occasionally, behaviours in toddlers may hint at issues like intussusception, urinary tract infections or minor injuries.

Seeking prompt medical advice when something seems unusual allows for appropriate intervention and helps maintain the child's health.

School-Age Children (4–12 years)

At this stage, children begin to describe their symptoms but cognitive and emotional 'immaturity' still colour their self-reporting. They may minimize, exaggerate or misunderstand their sensations.

Normal Responses	*Concerning Signs*
Vague complaints (for example, 'my tummy hurts') are often linked to stress or fatigue	Localized pain with functional limitation (for example, not walking due to limb pain)
Increased somatic complaints during transitions (for example, while starting school)	Night sweats, weight loss and persistent fever
Headaches, leg pains ('growing pains') or mild nausea without a clear cause	Recurrent or escalating complaints without an apparent cause

Appendicitis in children often begins with mild or vague abdominal discomfort that may gradually increase in the lower right abdomen and can be accompanied by tiredness or fever.

Because children may not always express their symptoms clearly, careful observation and timely medical evaluation are important. Early attention usually allows for straightforward treatment and prevents complications.

Interpreting 'Normal' vs 'Abnormal' in Context

The line between normal developmental behaviour and concerning body alarms is fluid. A tantrum can be a protest or a cry for help. Fatigue may follow a growth spurt or it may indicate anaemia or a chronic infection. Therefore, the context matters. The pattern, duration, intensity and change from the child's baseline are the key metrics.

A sudden shift in eating, sleeping or emotional tone should never be dismissed as 'just a phase' without considering the physiological underpinnings.

A child's body alarm, when correctly interpreted, may be the earliest clue to conditions ranging from infections or autoimmune disorders to abuse or emotional trauma.

Small Bodies, Strong Physical Signs

Children's bodies often manifest illness or internal distress before they can name it. Recognizing these physical alarms in visible, measurable changes is essential to timely intervention. Below are five of the most common body alarms that require careful attention and context-sensitive interpretation.

Fever and Unexplained Irritability

Fever is one of the most frequent symptoms in childhood and a well-known body alarm. While it's often the body's healthy response to infection, not all fevers are harmless. What raises concern is the context in which a fever occurs and what accompanies it. Irritability itself can be a stand-alone alarm.

For example, infants with middle-ear infections or toddlers with undiagnosed constipation may exhibit unusual fussiness long before any localized symptom appears. This behaviour is their body's way of signalling distress.

Changes in Breathing or Persistent Coughing

The respiratory system in children is more sensitive and narrower than in adults, which makes it prone to rapid decompensation.

Fast breathing, chest indrawing (when the ribs suck in during breaths), flaring nostrils and grunting sounds might signal pneumonia, bronchiolitis or even asthma in older children, sometimes.

A barking cough at night might indicate croup in some cases, while a whooping sound could point to pertussis.

What's alarming is that children may appear to be breathing 'okay' one minute and struggling the next. It's because their oxygen reserves are limited and their ability to compensate is short-lived.

Persistent coughing that disrupts sleep, is accompanied by vomiting, or produces coloured phlegm should always prompt evaluation.

Unusual Rashes or Skin Discolouration

Rashes in children are common. However, a non-blanching rash (that doesn't fade when pressed) may signal meningococcal infection, which can progress rapidly; sudden bruising or purpura (purple spots) without injury may reflect a clotting disorder; and pale, mottled or bluish skin may suggest circulation or oxygen problems.

More often, though, rashes stem from viral illnesses or allergies. In these cases, watch the context (for example, whether the child is itching severely and struggling to breathe, or if the rash is spreading quickly) to decide when medical care is needed.

Persistent Vomiting or Diarrhoea

Occasional vomiting or loose stools may come and go with viral bugs, but persistence changes the picture entirely. Dehydration is the real danger here, especially in infants and toddlers, whose fluid reserves are minimal.

Watch for dry lips, sunken eyes, lack of tears, reduced urination and lethargy. Repeated vomiting in the absence of fever or diarrhoea may point to surgical emergencies sometimes, like pyloric stenosis (in infants) or intestinal obstruction. Bloody stools or bile-stained vomit are also red flags that demand immediate attention.

These digestive symptoms shouldn't be ignored just because 'it happens to every child.'

Sudden Changes in Activity or Energy Levels

One of the most overlooked alarms is when a typically active child becomes listless, unusually still or uninterested in play. Children don't fake fatigue. If they stop engaging with their environment, it's often because something is wrong. Lethargy, unwillingness to sit up, difficulty keeping the eyes open or suddenly falling asleep in inappropriate settings may suggest serious infections, metabolic imbalances or internal injuries.

Even in less acute scenarios, a gradual but noticeable decline in activity over days or weeks may end up indicating chronic illnesses like anaemia, autoimmune disorders or undiagnosed diabetes.

It's important to distinguish between a tired child after a long day and one who shows a pattern of unexplained exhaustion. The body often slows down when it's fighting something invisible on the inside.

Kids' Behaviour Speaks Louder Than Words

While physical symptoms like fever or vomiting may prompt swift action, behavioural or emotional changes are often dismissed as phases or personality quirks. However, the body and mind are intricately linked, especially in children, where the line between emotional expression and physical discomfort is blurred.

Excessive Crying or Withdrawal

Crying is a child's first and most powerful language, but when crying becomes excessive, unprovoked or inconsolable, it may go beyond hunger or tiredness. In infants, sometimes crying intensifies simply when the mother or primary caregiver is absent. This is a normal developmental phase, especially between six months and three years, known as separation anxiety. It reflects the child's growing awareness of emotional attachment or fear of abandonment.

In older children, emotional withdrawal in forms such as sitting alone, avoiding interaction or disengaging from play may sometimes point towards chronic physical pain or anxiety that they cannot explain. Children at this age are often caught between developing self-awareness and a still-maturing emotional vocabulary.

Early recognition, patient listening and sensitive professional assessment can change the course of a child's emotional and physical development.

Changes in Sleep Patterns

Sleep is one of the clearest windows into a child's neurological and emotional health. Disruptions, such as excessive daytime sleepiness or night terrors, often reflect internal unrest.

Night waking in toddlers may signal teething, separation anxiety or even undiagnosed reflux.

Recurrent nightmares may result from overstimulation before bedtime or emotional stress that they cannot yet verbalize.

Excessive sleepiness in school-age children, especially when paired with lethargy, mood changes or poor school performance, may point to post-viral fatigue, early onset of depression or early signs of conditions like hypothyroidism or iron-deficiency anaemia.

In all cases, a sustained change in sleep behaviour, and not just one or two difficult nights, should be treated as a meaningful body alarm.

Keep a sleep diary for a week. Track bedtime, waking time, night wakings, naps and sleep quality. Note associated symptoms (for example, snoring, bedwetting and leg pain) and emotional patterns during the day.

Loss of Appetite or Refusal to Eat

Food refusal is often brushed off as fussiness, especially in toddlers. However, when eating habits change drastically, the body may be expressing discomfort. Gastrointestinal distress, mouth ulcers or infections can make eating painful. In older children, stress or anxiety may also suppress appetite subtly but significantly.

Persistent refusal to eat, especially when paired with weight loss or fatigue, may sometimes indicate serious underlying conditions as well, such as ARFID (avoidant/restrictive food intake disorder).

A child who stops eating is not always being 'difficult.'

They may be trying to tell you that something hurts or feels wrong inside. Pay attention.

Unusual Clinginess or Separation Anxiety

While some clinginess is developmentally normal, a sudden or intense need to stay physically close to a caregiver may signal fear, insecurity or even pain in some cases. Regressive clinginess in a previously independent child might sometimes follow an illness, a traumatic event or chronic discomfort. In younger children, excessive distress during separation may sometimes be the only behavioural sign of abdominal pain, headache or even urinary tract infections.

When this behaviour appears suddenly or persists beyond expected developmental phases, it's important to gently explore possible physical causes with a paediatrician, while also providing emotional reassurance through consistent routines and secure attachments.

Signs of Pain or Discomfort That Children Cannot Verbalize

Perhaps the most challenging body alarm is pain that a child cannot identify or describe. Instead of saying 'my leg hurts,' a toddler might stop walking. A school-aged child may refuse to participate in sports without being able to explain why.

Look for postural changes, facial grimaces, limping, the guarding of certain body parts and the avoidance of specific movements. Children may also show indirect signs like irritability, poor concentration or being quick to anger (unusual for their baseline temperament).

In one case, a six-year-old boy began refusing to sit during meals and had trouble sleeping. Weeks passed before an MRI revealed early spinal inflammation due to juvenile idiopathic arthritis (JIA).[20] Thus, his pain had a clear cause, but his behaviour was the only early alarm.

Recognizing Medical Emergencies

Children often recover quickly from minor ailments, but their bodies may also deteriorate just as fast when a serious condition is brewing. Timely recognition is crucial.

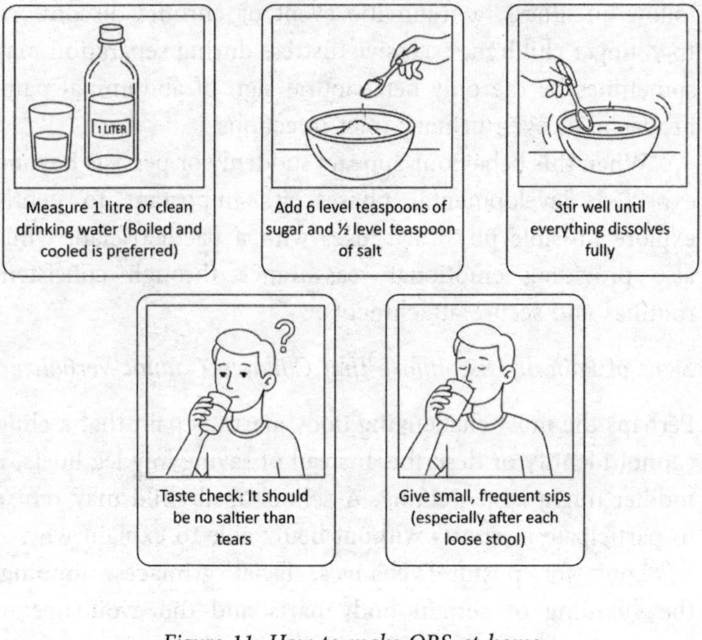

Figure 11: How to make ORS at home

[20]Ward, Teresa M., et al., 'Sleep Disturbances and Behaviour Problems in Children with and without Arthritis,' *Journal of Paediatric Nursing*, Vol. 29, No. 4, 2014), pp. 321–28.

Signs of Dehydration

Dehydration sometimes escalates rapidly in children, especially during vomiting, diarrhoea or high fevers. Because their bodies are smaller and water reserves are lower, even short-term fluid loss can become concerning. Watch for these signs:

- Dry mouth, sunken eyes, cool or mottled extremities
- No tears when crying
- Reduced urine output or dark-yellow urine
- Lethargy or listlessness

What to do: Encourage oral rehydration with electrolyte solutions. In moderate to severe cases, seek urgent care for IV fluids.

Seizures or Convulsions

A seizure is the brain's emergency flare, that is, electrical activity gone awry. While febrile seizures (triggered by high fever) are common in infants, any seizure should be evaluated, especially if prolonged or accompanied by unusual behaviour. Watch for these signs:

- Stiffening or jerking of limbs
- Loss of consciousness or staring spells
- Post-seizure confusion or deep sleep

What to do: Ensure that the child is lying safely on their side, and do not put anything in their mouth. Time the seizure. If it lasts more than five minutes, call emergency services immediately.

Difficulty Breathing or Choking

The inability to breathe properly is an immediate, life-threatening emergency. Children may struggle to describe breathlessness, but their bodies will show it. Watch for these signs:

- Rapid or laboured breathing
- Use of chest or neck muscles to breathe
- Gasping, grunting or wheezing
- Blue or greyish lips or fingertips

What to do: Administer prescribed inhalers (if available), use back blows if choking is suspected, and call emergency services without delay.

Sudden Limpness or Weakness

A child who suddenly goes limp, cannot stand or appears unusually weak may be experiencing a neurological or metabolic emergency. Even a brief episode of floppiness warrants evaluation.

Possible causes:

- Syncope (fainting)
- Low blood sugar
- Early signs of stroke (rare but possible)
- Neurological infections like encephalitis

What to do: Lay the child flat, ensure that the airway is clear and seek urgent medical help, especially if symptoms persist or are accompanied by vomiting or fever.

High Fever with Rash (Possible Meningitis)

A high fever alone is concerning, but as mentioned earlier, when paired with a new rash, it may signal meningitis or sepsis, both of which are potentially serious conditions. Watch for these signs:

- Purplish spots that don't blanch when pressed
- Stiff neck, light sensitivity or extreme irritability
- Confusion or difficulty waking the child

What to do: Don't wait. Go to the nearest emergency department, as timely care is key to effectively managing meningococcal infections.

Body Alarms in the Elderly

Physiological Changes with Ageing

Ageing alters the body's internal signalling systems. The same alarms that ring loudly in youth often soften, blur or shift pitch in older adults. This makes it particularly challenging to distinguish between what is expected and what is concerning.

Some physiological changes are part of healthy ageing:

- Reduced cardiac output and slightly elevated blood pressure
- Slower gastrointestinal motility
- Decreased bone density or muscle mass
- Mild memory lapses, such as forgetting names or misplacing objects
- Changes in sleep architecture, like lighter, shorter sleep cycles

However, these changes can sometimes mask or mimic the early signs of serious conditions.

For instance, mild forgetfulness may be normal, but forgetting recent events, repeating questions or disorientation could signal early cognitive decline. Likewise, fatigue and appetite loss may be attributed to ageing, but they are also hallmark symptoms of congestive heart failure, depression or malignancy.

Slower Symptom Onset and Atypical Presentations

Diseases that present with classic symptoms in younger people may emerge more subtly or misleadingly in older adults. This is especially true in infections, cardiovascular events and metabolic disorders. Consider these atypical presentations:

Urinary tract infections may cause confusion, agitation or falls without fever or pain.

Pneumonia may present as weakness or slight breathlessness rather than as a productive cough or high fever.

Myocardial infarctions in older adults often manifest as fatigue, indigestion or dizziness rather than chest pain.

Hyperthyroidism may look like weight loss or apathy (not tremors or anxiety).

The biological basis for this muted presentation lies in age-related changes to immune and nervous system responsiveness. Fever, inflammation and pain are often under-expressed. Sensory thresholds increase. Inflammatory cytokine response is slower. Neurological reflexes dampen.

This is why a seemingly minor symptom, like a new fall, unexplained tiredness or confusion, must not be brushed off in an elderly patient. These are often primary body alarms.

Common Physical Alarms in the Elderly

Sudden Weight Loss or Appetite Changes

Unintentional weight loss (for instance, more than five per cent of body weight over six to twelve months) is not a normal part of ageing. It often signals malignancy, thyroid disease, dementia or depression. In men, gastrointestinal cancers are a leading cause, and in women, autoimmune conditions or frailty syndromes may dominate.

Loss of appetite may also indicate early satiety from gastric motility issues or subtle signs of heart failure, where fluid overload suppresses hunger. Taste and smell also tend to decline with age, reducing food interest. This sensory loss is often compounded by loneliness, denture issues or even undiagnosed oral infections.

If a senior begins leaving meals untouched or loses noticeable weight without effort, investigate promptly.

Unexplained Pain or Chronic Discomfort

Pain in the elderly is underreported, often due to stoicism, fear of diagnosis or cognitive decline. However, failure to investigate pain properly may miss serious, treatable or even life-threatening conditions.

Persistent pain, especially if new or worsening, may sometimes point to degenerative joint disease, vascular insufficiency or even occult malignancy. Neuropathic pain, that is, burning, tingling or electric sensations, may reflect diabetic neuropathy or post-herpetic neuralgia. Generalized pain or discomfort may mask polymyalgia rheumatica, especially in women over sixty.

What to watch: Look for behavioural signs, such as guarding a limb, avoiding movement or grimacing during transfers, as many elders won't verbalize discomfort.

Changes in Mobility and Balance (Fall Risk)

Falls are among the most telling alarms in geriatrics and often the only symptom of a deeper issue. Even a single fall warrants assessment. It may point to orthostatic hypotension, polypharmacy, inner-ear dysfunction or visual impairment.

Vitamin D deficiency and declining proprioception tend to increase the risk in some cases.

Key insight: A fall is rarely 'just a fall.' It is the endpoint of a failing system (neuromuscular, cardiovascular or cognitive).

Evaluate for recent medication changes, check blood pressure in lying and standing positions, assess vision and refer for a comprehensive geriatric or physiotherapy balance assessment. Early intervention can prevent many complications like fractures, hospitalization or loss of independence.

Confusion or Sudden Cognitive Changes

Unlike dementia (which is gradual), delirium appears abruptly, often over hours to days. It is commonly triggered by infections (especially UTIs), medications, dehydration or metabolic imbalances. It may be the first or only symptom of pneumonia or sepsis in the elderly.

Sudden speech difficulty, facial droop and limb weakness must always be treated as a possible stroke. Silent strokes (affecting subcortical areas) may present as apathy, gait change or personality shifts without any dramatic paralysis.

Shortness of Breath or Chest Pain

In older adults, dyspnoea, even if mild, can sometimes indicate heart failure, pulmonary embolism or chronic obstructive pulmonary disease (COPD). Many elders don't describe 'pain' but rather 'pressure,' 'tightness,' or even 'just not feeling right.' In women, particularly, cardiac events may manifest as fatigue, nausea or light-headedness without chest pain at all.

Don't wait. Shortness of breath at rest or with minimal exertion should never be attributed solely to age or deconditioning.

Psychological and Cognitive Body Alarms

Depression, Anxiety, Social Isolation

Late-life depression is not sadness. It is often a slowing down of life. An older adult who stops participating in conversations, avoids hobbies or withdraws from social interactions may not be 'just tired.' Chronic anxiety can often appear as irritability, restlessness or complaints of vague physical symptoms. Social isolation itself, whether chosen or circumstantial, is both a symptom and a cause linked to higher mortality, cognitive decline or cardiovascular risk.

Early Signs of Dementia or Alzheimer's

Forgetfulness is not always benign. Misplacing objects, repeating questions or getting lost in familiar settings are early signs of neurodegenerative conditions like Alzheimer's. These may be brushed off as 'normal ageing' but timing and consistency matter. When forgetfulness begins interfering with daily function, it's no longer casual. Cognitive screening tools like the MMSE or MoCA should be used at this stage.

Sleep Disturbances or Excessive Fatigue

Frequent night waking, reversed sleep cycles or constant daytime drowsiness often precede psychological and neurological conditions. Sleep architecture changes with age but dramatic shifts, especially when paired with mood changes, may indicate depression, sleep apnoea or early dementia. Excessive fatigue can also be a masked symptom of chronic illness, heart failure or thyroid dysfunction sometimes.

Behavioural Changes Indicating Distress

A sudden loss of interest in grooming, increased suspicion,

hoarding behaviour or unexpected aggression should not be dismissed as 'old-age behaviour.' These may be expressions of fear, confusion or unspoken pain.

What to do: Early psychological intervention, cognitive assessment and a compassionate, structured routine can significantly delay progression and improve quality of life. Sometimes, quiet behaviour is the loudest alarm. Listen carefully.

Medication and Treatment-Related Alarms

In the elderly, medications are both a remedy and a risk. With age, the body's ability to metabolize and excrete drugs changes significantly. What was once a standard dose may now be too much or too little.

Adverse Drug Reactions or Side Effects

Older adults are more susceptible to drug side effects due to reduced kidney function, slower liver metabolism or polypharmacy. Common symptoms, including dizziness, confusion, constipation, tremors and gastrointestinal upset, may be brushed off as ageing but are often red flags of drug toxicity. For example, anticholinergic drugs (commonly found in over-the-counter sleep aids and allergy medications) can sometimes precipitate delirium or urinary retention in the elderly.

Non-Compliance or Misunderstanding Medication Instructions

Complex regimens with multiple pills, timing instructions and dietary restrictions can often lead to non-compliance not from neglect but from confusion. Vision problems, memory loss or hearing difficulties can all contribute to this. If a patient appears to worsen despite being 'on treatment,' the issue may sometimes lie in execution and not with the medication.

Signs of Withdrawal or Overdose

Missed doses of antidepressants, steroids or blood pressure medications can cause withdrawal symptoms in some cases, ranging from fatigue to severe mood changes or even cardiac events. On the other hand, overdosing, intentional or accidental, can be silent, especially with sedatives or pain medications. So, watch for excessive drowsiness, slowed breathing, slurred speech and unresponsiveness.

What to do: Medication reviews at regular intervals, especially during transitions of care, are essential. Involve pharmacists, simplify regimens and use pill organizers or digital reminders. In many cases, 'less is more' in geriatric pharmacology.

Recognizing Emergency Situations

In older adults, emergencies don't always announce themselves loudly. Age alters physiology, pain thresholds and symptom expression, thereby making early recognition a clinical and caregiving imperative.

Stroke Symptoms (FAST)

A stroke can be silent at first glance. Hence, use the FAST mnemonic:

F: Face drooping
A: Arm weakness
S: Speech slurring
T: Time to call emergency services

In the elderly, especially with silent strokes, symptoms may sometimes present as sudden confusion, imbalance or vision problems as well.

Heart Attack Signs

Chest pain may not be the leading symptom. Instead, look for jaw or shoulder discomfort, shortness of breath, cold sweats and unexplained fatigue. Diabetics and women in particular may present atypically with nausea, light-headedness or simply a 'sense of doom.'

Acute Infections (UTIs and Pneumonia)

Unlike younger individuals, elders may not spike fevers or show classic signs. A urinary tract infection may manifest as delirium or falls. Pneumonia may present only as lethargy or confusion. A sudden drop in function—that is, refusing food, missing medication and altered sleep—is often an infection in disguise.

Signs of Elder Abuse or Neglect

Unexplained bruises, burns, malnutrition, poor hygiene or fearful behaviour demand attention. Elder abuse can be physical, emotional, financial or medical, and it often hides in plain sight disguised as depression or decline. Trust your instinct when something feels 'off.'

What to do: Time matters. In all such alarms, act without delay. A prompt medical evaluation can mean the difference between full recovery and irreversible harm. In elder care, urgency must be guided not by volume of symptoms but by how quietly and subtly they appear.

A Listening Ear Mends More Than Medicine

Effective observation demands more than routine monitoring. It requires attentive, age-appropriate and empathetic communication. In children, this may mean reading the silence between words, interpreting play behaviour and watching how they cling or withdraw. In the elderly, it involves listening beyond complaints and recognizing when confusion replaces clarity or when subtle hesitation masks fear or fatigue.

Caregivers and professionals should maintain detailed, real-time symptom logs. A simple diary noting appetite, sleep, mood, mobility and unusual behaviours over days can reveal trends a single consultation may miss. Early documentation is often the key to connecting small signs before they become crises. Knowing when to escalate a low-grade fever with lethargy, a fall followed by confusion or a child's refusal to eat with signs of fatigue is as critical as identifying the symptoms themselves.

Preventive care plays an equally vital role. Regular health check-ups, developmental screenings in children and geriatric assessments in the elderly help identify silent changes before they become emergencies.

Families must be aware of what body alarms sound and look like at every age.

Empowered caregivers don't panic. They act!

Body Alarms in Those with Physical or Intellectual Disabilities

The human brain houses billions of neurons firing in an intricate dance, generating thoughts, sensations or alarms. In those with physical and intellectual disabilities, the body alarms demand new ways to listen beyond the obvious.

The body constantly sends signals to alert us about pain, discomfort or other changes that need attention. These 'body alarms' help us recognize when something is wrong and prompt us to take action. However, for people with physical or intellectual disabilities, these signals may not be felt clearly or may be difficult to express, making it harder to understand their needs and respond quickly.

In India, according to the 2011 Census, over 26.8 million people, that is about 2.2 per cent of the population, live with disabilities. More recent data from the National Family Health Survey-5 (NFHS-5, 2019–21) estimates a much higher prevalence of 4.52 per cent, totalling approximately 63.28 million people with disabilities.[21]

Many of these individuals have physical disabilities caused

---

[21]Pattnaik Sweta, Jogesh Murmu, Ritik Agrawal, Tanveer Rehman, Srikanta Kanungo, and Sanghamitra Pati, 'Prevalence, Pattern and Determinants of Disabilities in India: Insights from NFHS-5 (2019–21)', *Frontiers in Public Health*, Vol. 11, 2023, https://doi.org/10.3389/fpubh.2023.1036499. Accessed on 8 December 2025.

by injuries, neurological conditions or genetic disorders, which can affect their ability to feel pain or other important bodily sensations. For example, someone with a spinal cord injury (SCI) might not notice pressure sores developing, which can sometimes lead to serious infections if untreated. Similarly, intellectual disabilities, including conditions such as autism and developmental delays, can affect a person's ability to recognize or communicate their body's warning signs. Instead of saying they feel pain or discomfort, they may show distress through behaviour like agitation or withdrawal.

This chapter explores how body alarms work differently in people with physical or intellectual disabilities, what the challenges in detecting these signals are, and how important careful observation and communication are. It also discusses ways to improve detection through training, technology and teamwork among caregivers and professionals.

Physical Disabilities and the Body's Unedited Notes

Take cerebral palsy (CP) for example, where the brain's early injury scrambles the signals sent from limbs and muscles. Imagine a hand clenched tightly, rigid and aching, but the brain failing to register the sharpness of that pain. Or imagine the brain registering an overwhelming flood of sensation from a gentle touch that should be soothing. The mind and body fall out of sync and the person struggles to understand what their own body is telling them.

In spinal cord injury, it's as if the body below a certain point has been cut off from the world entirely. A burn or a deep cut might go unnoticed because the nerves that should scream 'danger!' are severed. This 'invisible' suffering demands constant vigilance from caregivers, for the individual can neither feel nor express the threat.

Further, muscular dystrophy brings a slow, creeping numbness. The muscles weaken, the posture falters and the internal cues signalling fatigue or distress become faint whispers drowned out by physical limitation. Famous individuals like Helen Keller and Stephen Hawking lived with such profound disruptions, yet they teach us how the human spirit endures.

How the Body's Alarms Break Down

Typically, sensory receptors detect threats in the form of heat that could burn, pressure that could bruise or a full bladder that demands relief, and they relay urgent messages through nerves to the brain. The brain deciphers these signals and initiates conscious awareness.

In physical disabilities, this chain breaks.

The brain misreads or dulls incoming sensory data. Automatic bodily responses like sweating to cool or shivering to warn of cold may be absent.

Learning to See the Invisible

Because the usual alarms may fail when it comes to physical disabilities, those who care must learn to see the invisible.

Vigilant observation becomes a lifeline (that is, checking skin for redness or swelling and noting changes in mood or breathing).

Communication aids and emergency readiness mean acting fast when subtle signs flare up.

Customized care such as pressure relief devices or scheduled health checks prevents hidden harms.

To live with a disrupted body alarm is to navigate a world where pain and danger hide beneath the surface. Nevertheless, it all gets easier with understanding, empathy and attentive care.

Body Responses in Intellectual Disabilities

Now, suppose you wake up one morning with a strange sensation inside your body but you have no words for it and no way to say what you feel. You only know something is wrong. You cry, lash out, go silent or rock back and forth… anything to make the discomfort leave or be understood.

This is not a rare experience. For millions of individuals with intellectual disabilities, this is how their body's alarm system works: unclear, misunderstood and often ignored.

Understanding Intellectual Disabilities

Intellectual disabilities are characterized by limitations in cognitive functioning and adaptive behaviour. Conditions such as autism spectrum disorder (ASD), Down syndrome and global developmental delay (GDD) affect how individuals learn, communicate and relate to their environment, including how they perceive or respond to body signals.

Unlike physical disabilities, the issue is not necessarily in the reception of signals from the body but in the interpretation and communication of those signals. A headache may be experienced as intense confusion. A stomach ache might trigger sudden aggression. Hunger could lead to withdrawal or crying.

Every internal sensation travels through a mind that might not have the words, logic or emotional regulation tools to explain it.

Difficulties in Recognition and Communication

The challenge is twofold:

Recognition of Internal Cues: Many individuals with intellectual disabilities struggle to identify or differentiate between bodily sensations. Pain, discomfort, fatigue or hunger may feel overwhelming or diffuse, making it difficult to label or localize.

Expression of Discomfort: Instead of verbal complaints, distress may appear in behaviour in the form of self-injury, aggression, screaming, running away or even complete withdrawal. These are not acts of defiance. The behaviour is the language.

For example, a child with autism might bang their head repeatedly because it's the only way they know how to show that something feels wrong. And a teenager with Down syndrome might refuse to eat because of a toothache they cannot describe.

These expressions are often misread as behavioural problems (such as 'stubbornness') when they are, in fact, body alarms most of the time.

The Role of Caregivers and Professionals

Here, caregivers and professionals are interpreters as well as supporters. They must learn the language of behaviour to understand that a sudden change in mood, activity or expression might indicate a fever, constipation, pain or anxiety too. Tools and strategies include:

Behavioural Tracking: Monitoring patterns can reveal links between physical states and outbursts or shutdowns.

Visual Aids and Pain Scales: Simplified communication tools such as face charts and colour-coded cards can help individuals indicate how they feel.

Training in Emotional Literacy: Helping individuals name and understand feelings or sensations fosters independence and safety.

Tech Strategies for Better Detection

Technology has the potential to compensate where biology lags. Innovative tools can monitor internal states, translate discomfort into data and alert caregivers before a situation escalates. For persons who cannot verbalize their needs, these devices become the mediators of experience.

Wearable Health Monitors

Devices that continuously track physiological indicators such as heart rate variability, skin conductance, temperature, oxygen saturation and movement patterns can help identify early signs of distress, pain, fatigue or even emotional dysregulation.

Smart Alarms and Sensors

Posture monitors and pressure-mapping sensors embedded in wheelchairs, cushions and beds detect when a person hasn't moved and issue reminders or alerts, which are crucial for those with reduced mobility who are at risk of pressure ulcers or circulatory issues. Smart mattresses and bedding systems can automatically adjust pressure zones, thereby reducing the need for manual repositioning and increasing user comfort.

Adaptive Communication Devices (AAC)

These include speech-generating devices, picture-based apps, eye-tracking tablets and gesture-recognition software (that translates movements into digital input). These tools help users express basic needs, report discomfort and request help.

AI-Powered Behavioural Analytics

Some platforms now use machine learning to detect patterns of distress from audio, facial expression and movement, which is especially useful for people with severe intellectual disabilities. AI can flag anomalies faster than humans, such as changes in tone, facial micro-expressions and motion rhythms that precede a meltdown or medical issue.

Environmental Sensing Systems

Integrated IoT (Internet of Things) systems in smart homes or care facilities help monitor temperature, air quality, light and noise levels. For individuals sensitive to sensory input (such as those with autism), these environments can be adapted automatically to prevent distress.

Biofeedback and Neurofeedback Devices

These tools give users and caregivers real-time feedback about stress or physiological arousal. Wearable EEGs or skin conductance monitors can detect rising anxiety levels and allow for calming interventions before full escalation.

Emergency Response Wearables

Wristbands or pendants with fall detection, SOS buttons and GPS tracking provide safety, especially for those with limited speech or a high risk of seizures or injury.

Having said that, technology should not replace human attentiveness. Instead, it should augment it to support faster, more informed and more dignified interventions.

Designing 'With,' Not 'For'

Helen Keller's first word wasn't spoken. It was felt. When her teacher spelt 'water' into her hand under a running pump, language, once trapped inside her, surged outward. A century later, Stephen Hawking's cheek muscle controlled a computer that spoke entire words. However, that system also worked only because it was designed with him. It learned his pace, his fatigue and his way of saying 'yes' when the rest of his body said nothing.

Today, as we strive to understand body alarms in persons with disabilities, we must remember that the most advanced tool is useless if it doesn't fit the person.

In the end, it is not just about being high-tech.

It is about being human-aware.

The Prelude to Mental Illness

'Voices echo in my head, but they don't speak words. They press on me with feelings I can't explain. Colours seem sharper, shadows twist oddly and sometimes my own hands feel foreign like they are moving on their own. My heart races for no reason I can name, and my muscles tense as if I am preparing to run from something I can't see. I am awake, but parts of me drift away, perhaps caught between reality and something else.'

Psychiatrists and psychologists study the mind, but most have never lived inside these kinds of experiences, which often combine the swirling confusion, the sensory overload and the constant tension between reality and hallucination. They rely on observations and clinical frameworks to make sense of what is an overwhelming flood of fragmented perceptions or bodily signals that cannot be easily described as a restless pulse, a creeping numbness or an unexplained ache.

For someone without training or insight, these early signs are even harder to recognize. The body's subtle alarms get dismissed as stress or tiredness. Without understanding, confusion deepens. The person struggles alone, caught between internal chaos and external misunderstanding. The gap tends to widen, symptoms tend to worsen, and fear tends to grow of being judged, misunderstood or dismissed entirely.

Many of us have lost dear friends, family members or colleagues to these battles. Their struggles often began with these alarms we failed to hear. You yourself might be experiencing these signs right now without even realizing it.

This chapter is a call to listen closely to the body's early warnings and to learn a new language of mental illness.

When Your Mind Isn't Playing by the 'Rules,' Your Body Sounds a Different Alarm

When you think of mental illness, you might picture something happening solely inside the mind. However, your body and mind are in constant communication, exchanging signals that influence how you feel, think and behave. This ongoing dialogue is complex but essential to understanding early signs of mental distress.

Take the gut-brain connection, for example.[22] Your gut is often called your 'second brain' because it contains millions of nerve cells and produces about 90 per cent of your body's serotonin, which is a key chemical that regulates mood. The trillions of bacteria living in your intestines also play a surprising role and affect the balance of brain chemicals linked to anxiety, depression or even conditions like schizophrenia. Studies have found that people with mental health challenges often have different gut bacteria than those without, suggesting that your digestive system and mental health may be more closely linked than is acknowledged.[23]

---

[22]Mayer, Emeran, *The Mind-Gut Connection: How the Hidden Conversation within Our Bodies Impacts Our Mood, Our Choices, and Our Overall Health*, Harper Wave, New York, 2016.

[23]Grau-Del Valle, C.G., Javier Fernández, Eva Solá, Inmaculada Montoya-Castilla, Carlos Morillas, and Celia Bañuls, 'Association between Gut Microbiota and Psychiatric Disorders', *Frontiers in Psychology*, Vol. 14, 2023, https://doi.org/10.3389/fpsyg.2023.1215674. Accessed on 8 December 2025.

Then, there is your autonomic nervous system (ANS), which controls automatic functions like your heart rate and breathing. When you feel stressed or anxious, the ANS triggers a 'fight or flight' response, where your heart races, muscles tighten and stress hormones flood your system. While this response is helpful in short bursts, constant activation can sometimes harm brain areas responsible for memory, emotion and decision-making, and make you more vulnerable to anxiety or depression.

Your immune system also plays a role in this conversation. Chronic inflammation, which is the body's prolonged immune response, releases chemicals that can disrupt brain function and mood regulation, thus further linking physical health with mental well-being.

Understanding this intimate mind-body dialogue empowers you to respond to mental distress with greater awareness and compassion, both for yourself and for others.

The Mind–Body Dialogue

Depression: 'Can't Find the Energy Even to Try'

You wake up drained, though the night passed quietly. You move slowly, as if gravity has doubled overnight. Your appetite has changed. Maybe food repels you or maybe it's the only thing that offers comfort. Sleep, once peaceful, becomes either evasive or excessive. You cannot think clearly, and your body aches in ways doctors can't explain.

This is how depression often begins.

Depression is traditionally thought of as a mental illness, but in truth, it is often deeply physical. More than two-thirds of patients with depression are said to report only somatic symptoms, indicating that the body's complaints appear before any emotional distress is recognized.[24] These can include:

- Persistent fatigue, even after rest
- Unexplained muscle or joint pain
- Digestive disturbances, like constipation or nausea
- Weight fluctuations due to appetite changes
- Disordered sleep
- Reduced libido (which can be an early hormonal indicator)
- Tension headaches (particularly in women)

These symptoms aren't side effects. They are often the main effects. And still, people tend to dismiss them as stress, lifestyle or ageing.

Depression Wears a Body

Sometimes, depression wears the body like a shroud. In psychomotor retardation, everything slows. A person may speak more softly, walk more slowly and struggle to initiate tasks. It's as if the mind and body are disconnected. Thoughts become sluggish and even brushing your teeth feels monumental.

On the other end, some experience psychomotor agitation. They can't sit still. Fingers twitch, legs bounce and pacing becomes habitual. There is internal chaos and a restlessness that has nowhere to go.

These motor symptoms are often misread as laziness or anxiety. However, they are physical manifestations of a deeply distressed nervous system.

---

[24]Tylee, André, and Paul Gandhi, 'The Importance of Somatic Symptoms in Depression in Primary Care', *Primary Care Companion to the Journal of Clinical Psychiatry*, Vol. 7, No. 4, 2005, pp. 167–176, https://doi.org/10.4088/pcc.v07n0405. Accessed on 8 December 2025.

The Role of the Immune System

We usually separate physical and mental health but your immune system doesn't. Depression is thus increasingly seen as a systemic condition where low-grade chronic inflammation contributes to fatigue, pain, brain fog or emotional blunting. Inflammatory markers like C-reactive protein (CRP) and interleukin-6 (IL-6) are often elevated in people with depression even when they appear physically healthy.[25]

All this may explain why depression is so common among those with autoimmune disorders or chronic illnesses and why it often coexists with seemingly unrelated physical conditions.

What Can Be Done

When physical symptoms persist without a clear medical cause, consult both a primary care physician and a mental health professional. A multidisciplinary approach, which combines medical evaluation, psychotherapy, lifestyle interventions and, where appropriate, pharmacological support, often proves most effective.

Anxiety Disorders: 'Why Can't I Just Relax?'

What if the danger is imagined but the body reacts as if it's real? For many, anxiety doesn't begin as a thought. It begins as a flutter in the chest, a cold sweat or a stomach that clenches without warning. Long before the mind recognizes panic, the

---

[25]Osimo, Emanuele Felice, Luke James Baxter, Glyn Lewis, Peter B. Jones, and Golam M. Khandaker, 'Prevalence of Low-Grade Inflammation in Depression: A Systematic Review and Meta-Analysis of CRP Levels', *Psychological Medicine*, Vol. 49, No. 12, 2019, pp. 1958–70, https://doi.org/10.1017/s0033291719001454. Accessed on 8 December 2025.

body races ahead, primed for danger that may never arrive.

Anxiety disorders are deeply embodied experiences. The body's alarm system, which is meant to protect against real threats, goes into overdrive, responding to internal fears as though they were external attacks. At the heart of anxiety lies a nervous system on high alert. The autonomic nervous system, especially the sympathetic branch, controls involuntary functions like heartbeat, breathing, digestion and sweating. When anxiety takes hold, this system ramps up.

Common symptoms include:

- Racing or irregular heartbeat
- Shortness of breath or hyperventilation
- Sweating (even in cool temperatures)
- Dry mouth or a choking sensation
- Trembling or shakiness

These symptoms reflect a fight-or-flight response, often activated by perceived threat. For someone with generalized anxiety, social anxiety or panic disorder, this state can often become the default, leaving the body perpetually exhausted or overstimulated.

Muscle Tension, Headaches and Chronic Strain

Anxiety often lodges itself in the muscles. People with anxiety frequently experience:

- Tightness in the shoulders, neck and jaw
- Frequent tension headaches
- Teeth grinding (especially during sleep)
- Lower back pain or general body soreness

This constant physical strain can lead to misdiagnoses in the form of chronic migraines, TMJ disorders or even fibromyalgia in some cases when the root cause is ongoing, unrecognized anxiety.

The Gut as a Battlefield

The gut-brain axis plays a major role in anxiety, where emotional distress often disrupts digestion and gut motility. For some, this presents as:

- Symptoms similar to irritable bowel syndrome (IBS)
- Nausea or appetite suppression
- Bloating or gas
- Frequent need to use the restroom before or during anxiety-provoking situations

These symptoms are real. The brain and gut share a bidirectional connection and during anxious episodes, gastrointestinal function is one of the first systems to react.

Panic Attacks: 'My Chest Feels Tight, Like I Can't Breathe!'

A panic attack is a sudden surge of overwhelming fear, and it is so intense that it can feel like a heart attack or even dying. While panic attacks are psychological in origin, their presentation is almost entirely physical. Typical signs include:

- Chest pain or tightness
- Pounding heart (palpitations)
- Shortness of breath or a choking feeling
- Dizziness, light-headedness or feeling faint
- Hot flashes or chills
- Numbness or tingling in the hands or face
- A feeling of unreality (derealization)

Many people first encounter mental health services not through a psychologist but in an emergency room, terrified that they are having a cardiac event. It's only after repeated 'all-clear' results that anxiety is considered.

Anxiety Mimics Physical Illnesses

Anxiety can frequently imitate the symptoms of serious medical conditions. For example, chest pain mimics angina, shortness of breath mimics asthma, muscle tension mimics neurological issues, and dizziness and fatigue mimic anaemia or thyroid problems.

All this leads to frequent doctor visits, endless diagnostic tests and mounting frustration. For some, the medical odyssey delays effective mental health intervention.

What Can Be Done

Effective treatment of anxiety must address both mind and body. Cognitive-behavioural therapy (CBT) helps reframe catastrophic thoughts. Mindfulness practices help regulate the nervous system. In some cases, medications such as SSRIs or beta-blockers provide essential support. Equally important are lifestyle interventions echoed in nutrition, sleep hygiene, breathwork and movement, tailored to soothe a body dealing with anxiety.

Bipolar Disorder: 'One Day I'm on Top of the World, the Next I'm in a Hole'

More often, bipolar disorder enters the body first through sudden restlessness, boundless energy or profound fatigue that sleep cannot cure. The condition is commonly associated with alternating manic and depressive states.

During manic or hypomanic phases, individuals may feel physically invincible, needing less sleep, moving constantly, pacing, gesturing with speed and even engaging in risky physical activity. Appetite may plummet and the body seems to run on an invisible fuel. During depressive episodes, on the other hand, the opposite is true. Movement slows, limbs feel heavy, and even basic tasks like bathing or walking may become overwhelming.

These energy shifts are somatic reflections of biochemical mood changes.

Recognizing the Body's Subtle Cues

Sleep disturbances are among the most reliable early warning signs of a mood shift for those living with bipolar disorder and for the professionals or caregivers supporting them. Reduced need for sleep and feeling rested after only a few hours or skipping sleep altogether can indicate an oncoming manic phase. Conversely, oversleeping, insomnia or irregular sleep-wake patterns often accompany depressive phases.

Further, physical expressions of mood are subtle but telling.

- Rapid, pressured speech
- Restless pacing or fidgeting
- Hand tremors from increased psychomotor activity
- Dramatic changes in clothing, posture or grooming

During manic states, individuals may feel physically powerful, leading to increased sexual activity, excessive exercise or impulsive travel. Conversely, depressive states can bring slumped posture, a blank gaze, minimal facial expression and psychomotor retardation, where the body itself seems slowed down.

What Can Be Done

Bipolar disorder can be profoundly destabilizing, but body awareness can offer grounding. Identifying early physical signs such as sleep disruptions, energy surges or collapses and bodily agitation allows for timely therapeutic adjustments. Stabilizing routines around sleep, movement and nourishment are essential. Treatment plans that combine mood stabilizers, psychotherapy and somatic awareness techniques (such as yoga, breathwork and sensory tracking) empower individuals to anticipate and navigate mood shifts more effectively.

Mood diaries that include physical sensations, sleep data and activity levels are often more revealing than mood descriptions alone.

Schizophrenia and Associated Psychotic Conditions: 'My Mind Doesn't Belong to Me Sometimes

Schizophrenia is often imagined as a condition of hallucinations and delusions. However, the journey towards psychosis rarely begins with voices or paranoia. Long before the first psychotic break, the body often shows signs that something is changing.[26]

Common prodromal physical symptoms include:

- Sensory distortions (heightened sensitivity to light, sound, touch or smell)
- Changes in movement (mild coordination issues, awkward gait or clumsiness)
- Strange bodily sensations (feeling detached from limbs or sensations of heaviness or lightness)
- Fatigue or diminished physical motivation

These signs may appear months or even years before clinical diagnosis. While subtle, they suggest an altered integration of perception, movement and bodily control, which are core

[26]Fusar-Poli, Paolo, et al., 'The Psychosis High-Risk State: A Comprehensive State-of-the-Art Review', *JAMA Psychiatry*, Vol.70, No. 1, 2013, pp. 107–120.

components of schizophrenia's neurological disruption.

Schizophrenia often unravels the body's most basic rhythms as well. Key early disturbances include:

- Insomnia or reversed sleep-wake cycles (often appearing before psychosis)
- Nightmares or vivid dreams that feel intensely real
- Loss of appetite or binge-eating episodes (often disconnected from emotional context)
- Weight loss or gain in the absence of a clear cause

These changes are deep disruptions in hypothalamic regulation, which controls circadian rhythms, hunger cues and stress responses.

What Can Be Done

In cases of suspected psychotic illness, early detection is key. Structured screening for prodromal signs, attention to physical changes and swift referral to a mental health professional can alter the trajectory of the condition.

When schizophrenia is identified early and treated as a whole-body illness, outcomes tend to improve dramatically. Encouraging psychoeducation, routine physical check-ups and movement-based therapies (such as physiotherapy and dance therapy) can reconnect the patient with the physical self, which is often the first part of the story to go unheard.

PTSD: 'My Body Bolts Before My Mind Understands Why'

Trauma doesn't end when the event does. For many, the real impact begins long after the danger has passed and when the body can't seem to return to safety.

PTSD (post-traumatic stress disorder) and other trauma-related disorders are not simply conditions of memory or mood. They are embodied experiences. The body, in its need to survive, often holds the story of trauma long after the mind has tried to forget it.

Chronic Pain, Muscle Tightness and Somatic Complaints

Many individuals with PTSD live with persistent, unexplained physical pain. Neck and back pain, migraines and digestive issues are among the most reported complaints.[27] Muscle tightness, particularly in the shoulders, jaw and abdomen, is also common and is part of a body braced for impact long after the threat is gone.

Further, the body remembers trauma in muscle tone, in posture and even in how one breathes. These physical states often form, without conscious awareness, as protective mechanisms that no longer serve their original purpose.

Fibromyalgia-like symptoms, fatigue and general physical discomfort often coexist with trauma, though they may not be immediately linked.

Hypervigilance in the Flesh

Trauma heightens the body's alarm system, especially the amygdala and autonomic nervous system. As a result, hypervigilance is intensely physical as well as psychological. Common physical expressions include:

- A racing heart even at rest
- Startle reflexes triggered by ordinary sounds or movements

[27]Mayer, Emeran A., 'Somatic Manifestations of Traumatic Stress', in *Understanding Trauma: Integrating Biological, Clinical, and Cultural Perspectives*, Laurence J. Kirmayer, Robert Lemelson, and Mark Barad (eds.), Cambridge University Press, Cambridge, 2007, pp. 142–170.

- Sweating, shaking or freezing in response to perceived danger
- Tight fists, grinding teeth or scanning movements that indicate constant alertness

These reactions are part of the body's attempt to protect itself. However, over time, they exhaust the system, disrupting daily functioning and physical health.

Flashbacks and Their Physiological Echoes

Flashbacks are full-body experiences and often outside conscious control. During a flashback, the body may:

- React as if the traumatic event is happening again
- Experience increased heart rate, rapid breathing, trembling, nausea or muscle collapse
- Lose track of time and physical surroundings

Prolonged or severe trauma thus recalibrates the body's entire defence mechanism. The nervous system becomes sensitized and reacts strongly even to non-threatening stimuli sometimes.

What Can Be Done

Recovery from trauma is about processing memories and rebuilding trust between the body and the self. Effective approaches often include:

- Somatic therapies like EMDR (eye movement desensitization and reprocessing), sensorimotor psychotherapy and somatic experiencing
- Breathwork, yoga, and trauma-informed physical practices that allow the body to regulate and release
- Safe, predictable routines to signal safety to the nervous system

- Touch therapies and grounding exercises to re-anchor the body in the present

These practices are 'wellness tools' as well as interventions that target the body's alarm systems directly.

OCD: 'My Rituals Feel Like Rules I Can't Break'

For someone living with obsessive-compulsive disorder (OCD), thoughts do not simply visit the mind. Rather, they lodge there, looping endlessly and demanding action. And often, it's the body that is conscripted to carry out these compulsive orders, sometimes hundreds of times a day. While OCD is typically understood as a mental condition, it manifests intensely through physical behaviours by means of rituals, repetitions and routines that may exhaust or even injure the body.

Physical Rituals and Compulsions

In OCD, compulsions are physical responses to mental distress. These are not simply habits or quirks but actions performed to neutralize, suppress or prevent feared events.

Examples include:

- Hand-washing rituals that go far beyond hygiene
- Lock-checking, counting or tapping to create a sense of control
- Repetitive cleaning, rearranging or checking behaviours

Each action provides momentary relief from obsessive thoughts, but the repetition itself becomes a burden, often consuming hours and stripping away physical ease.

Over time, these compulsive movements may cause:

- Skin damage (for example, cracked or bleeding hands from over-washing)

- Joint strain or repetitive stress injuries from repeated physical motions
- Muscle fatigue, particularly in the back, shoulders and arms
- Headaches and jaw tension from grinding teeth or clenching under stress

Related Conditions and Their Physical Expressions

OCD is part of a broader family of obsessive-compulsive and related disorders, including:

- Body dysmorphic disorder (BDD) (which leads to excessive grooming, skin picking or mirror checking)
- Trichotillomania (compulsive hair pulling, which can result in bald patches, skin infections or shame)
- Excoriation disorder (skin picking that leads to scarring or dermatological damage)
- Hoarding disorder (though less physically repetitive, it often causes chronic stress, poor posture and physical strain from navigating cluttered unsafe spaces)

These conditions often involve physical rituals and behaviours tied to distressing thoughts, making them bodily disorders as much as psychological ones.

What Can Be Done

Helping someone with OCD isn't about telling them to 'just stop.' It is about understanding that their body is speaking a language of fear and seeking relief in repetitive rituals.

Recognizing OCD and related disorders early requires looking beyond the mind and watching the body and noticing the rubbed-raw hands, the constant fidgeting and the exhausted posture. Effective treatment often includes cognitive behavioural therapy (CBT), particularly exposure and response prevention (ERP), alongside SSRIs and body-oriented therapies.

Communicating Compassionately about Body Alarms

For centuries, those labelled 'mentally unwell' were bound to ships, with their fate cast to the uncertain seas. These vessels became floating prisons that carried souls misunderstood, feared and accused of witchcraft or demonic possession.[28]

How we speak to others and to ourselves can determine whether suffering stays hidden or begins to heal. Recognizing physical signs of mental distress is an essential step. Whether supporting someone we love or navigating our own private storm, compassion is the bridge that makes healing possible.

Principles of Compassionate Communication

Mental illness is often entangled with shame, confusion and fear. This makes communication a delicate terrain. A dismissive comment or a rushed interpretation can unintentionally reinforce withdrawal. Conversely, a well-placed, gentle question can invite openness. These approaches help foster trust, clarity and emotional safety:

> *Speak in terms of concern, not correction.*
> Show care without sounding accusatory.
> Say: 'I have noticed you seem more tired than usual. How have you been feeling?'
> Not: 'You are always sleeping. What is wrong with you?'

[28]'Prison Hulks', *Convicts Research Guide*, National Library of Australia, https://tinyurl.com/7jhsx45k. Accessed on 8 December 2025.

Focus on the body.

It is often easier to begin with the physical.

'You have been mentioning headaches a lot. Do you think it might be related to stress or something else?'

Offer presence, not pressure.

Allow space and time, without forcing a response.

'I am here for you. You don't have to explain everything now. When you are ready, I will listen.'

Avoid armchair diagnoses.

Resist the urge to name or interpret someone's condition prematurely.

'I have noticed a few things changing. Would you be open to exploring this with someone qualified?'

Extending This Compassion Inward

How we speak to ourselves is just as important as anything else we do. Internal self-talk, especially during distress, can be critical or kind, and the difference matters.

Instead of: 'Why can't I just snap out of this?'

Try: 'Something in me needs care. Can I slow down and listen?'

Having said that, compassionate communication, external or internal, is not about having perfect words. It is about being willing to witness discomfort without judgement, to create space without rushing in to fix, and to remind ourselves and others that you are not alone and your experience matters.

Developing this inner dialogue of empathy is the foundation of self-awareness and healing. Body alarms are easier to ignore when we have silenced ourselves for too long.

'I See Dead People...'

In the movie *The Sixth Sense*, a young boy famously confesses, 'I see dead people.' At first, his visions are dismissed as hallucinations or signs of mental illness, but as the story unfolds, it becomes clear that what he experiences is something beyond conventional understanding. There is thus a blurred line between psychological distress and the supernatural. This haunting ambiguity often challenges us to reconsider how we interpret unusual mental experiences.

From a scientific perspective, hallucinations and altered perceptions arise from complex neurobiological processes and involve imbalances in brain chemistry, disruptions in neural circuits or heightened activity in sensory processing areas. However, science also acknowledges the limits of current understanding about consciousness and subjective experience. This leaves room for questions about the nature of reality as perceived by the mind and reminds us that some phenomena do resist simple classification.

Nonetheless, though we may never fully unravel the blurred line between mind and mystery or between illness and insight, what can be done is to remain vigilant, to listen carefully to our body's alarms, and to respond with awareness rather than fear.

In this mindful attention lies the possibility of early intervention and a deeper connection to ourselves.

PART 3

THE BODY'S SECRETIONS AND SIGNALS

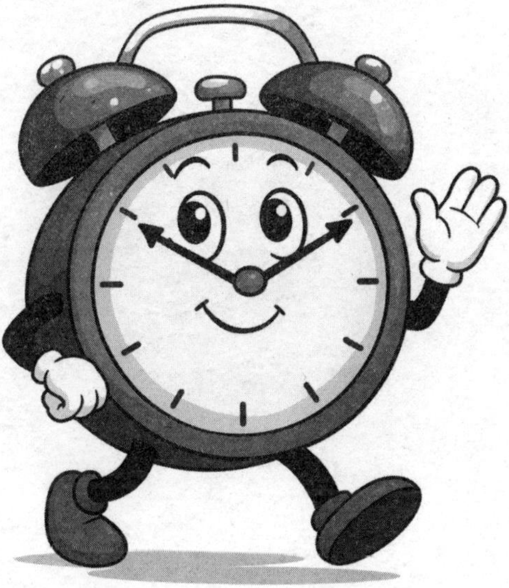

To Understand Your Fluids Is to Understand Your Body's Inner Logic

From the amniotic sac that shields your first breath to the blood that sustains each heartbeat, your existence is immersed, quite literally, in liquid. Thus, your body is not a machine of rigid parts, but instead, it's a dynamic ecosystem where fluids carry oxygen, relay signals, dissolve nutrients and remove waste.

As you go about your day, a slight change in the smell of your sweat, a new hue in your urine or the texture of your phlegm may seem unimportant. However, to the trained eye, and increasingly to those who learn to listen, these changes can sometimes mark the difference between early detection and late diagnosis.

Still, culturally and socially, bodily fluids are frequently met with discomfort, silence or even shame. We conceal stains, mask smells, and rarely ask questions despite the fact that these fluids often tell us what no scan or test does in the earliest stages.

In this chapter, we will explore the language of bodily fluids with respect to what they are made of, why they appear and what they mean.

Just as engineers read gauges or pilots scan dashboards, you, too, will read the signs your body presents.

Understanding the ABCs of Bodily Fluids

In space missions, survival depends on noticing the smallest deviations such as a hiss of escaping gas or a film of moisture where none should be.

A bodily fluid is any liquid produced by the body that plays a role in sustaining life, maintaining balance or expelling waste. While the term may evoke only blood or urine at first, the human body produces a wide spectrum of fluids, some of which are visible and others microscopic, some continuous and others situational.

Far from being inert waste, bodily fluids are alive with purpose. They contain cells, enzymes, hormones, antibodies, electrolytes and microbiota, making them a treasure trove for understanding how the body communicates, protects and adapts.

What Flows inside You?

To make sense of their roles, bodily fluids can be broadly categorized into secretions, excretions and emissions.

Secretions are fluids produced and retained within the body to perform specific functions. They are usually active agents in internal processes. Examples include saliva (which begins digestion and contains antimicrobial agents), mucus (which traps pathogens and lubricates passages), gastric juices (which aid digestion and regulate stomach acidity) and tears (which lubricate and cleanse the eyes).

Excretions are fluids that the body produces to eliminate waste or excess. Their removal is essential to maintaining internal balance. Examples include urine (which removes urea and toxins and regulates hydration), sweat (which aids thermoregulation and excretes salts) and faeces (which expel indigestible material and gut flora byproducts).

Finally, emissions are fluids associated with reproductive and sexual functions, often carrying biological material for potential fertilization. Examples include semen (which transports sperm), vaginal discharge (which protects and maintains vaginal health) and breast milk (which nourishes and immunologically protects infants).

The Many Faces of Bodily Fluids

First, There Are the Eyes...

Basal, Emotional and Reflex Tears

Tears are not all the same. Though they may look alike, they are produced under different circumstances and with distinct biochemical compositions.

Basal tears are a constant, nourishing layer (rich in enzymes, lipids and electrolytes) which keeps the eyes lubricated and the vision clear. Reflex tears spring forth in response to irritants like dust, smoke or onion vapours, flushing out foreign particles with a mostly watery composition. Emotional tears, triggered by intense feelings, carry stress-related hormones such as ACTH and hint at a fascinating link between our physiological responses and emotional well-being.

Knowing about these tears helps us understand eye function, recognize warning signs of eye problems, and appreciate the connection between our body and emotions.

The Sticky Stuff

Ocular discharge, particularly upon waking, is usually composed of dried mucus, oils, skin cells and dust, and is benign in small amounts.

However, when discharge becomes excessive, yellow-green or foul-smelling, it may sometimes indicate:

- Bacterial or viral conjunctivitis (commonly known as pink eye)
- Blocked tear ducts (especially in infants or ageing adults)
- Blepharitis (that is, an inflammation of the eyelid margins)
- Allergic conjunctivitis (which typically presents with clear or stringy mucus and is often accompanied by intense itching)

Distinguishing between infectious and allergic discharge is key.

Bacterial infections usually produce thick, coloured pus and may affect one eye first. Allergies, on the other hand, typically affect both eyes symmetrically and involve more itching than pain.

Nasal Drip and Mucus Explained

Colours and Consistency

Nasal mucus changes in colour, volume and viscosity (depending on what your body is going through).

Colour	*Consistency*	*Likely Cause*	*What It May Be Telling You*
Clear	Thin and watery mucus	May indicate normal function or allergies	Either all is well or it's a small reaction to irritants or allergens.

Colour	*Consistency*	*Likely Cause*	*What It May Be Telling You*
White/ cloudy	Thickened mucus	Often indicates nasal inflammation or an early viral infection	Congestion may be building, so it's wise to take early steps to relieve it.
Yellow	Sticky and thick mucus	Signals a progressing viral infection	The immune system is fighting. Monitor for worsening symptoms, if any.
Green	Dense and opaque mucus	May indicate a viral or bacterial infection	The immune response is intensifying, and it could signal the need for medical review.
Red/brown	Blood-tinged mucus	Often due to irritated or dry nasal tissue	May indicate mucosal injury. Consider hydration or gentler care.
Black	Mucus of variable consistency	May indicate a fungal infection or toxin exposure	Although rare, this is serious and requires immediate medical attention.

Allergies vs Infections

Never assume that every runny nose is just a cold or a seasonal allergy. Here's how to tell what may need urgent care.

Allergic Rhinitis	*Viral Infection*	*Bacterial Infection*
Clear mucus, frequent sneezing and itchy eyes	Begins with clear mucus that may turn yellow or green	Persistent thick green or yellow discharge (lasting more than 10 days)
No fever	May involve low-grade fever and body aches	Accompanied by facial pain, pressure, bad breath or fever
Triggered by pollen, dust or dander	Usually self-limited, but requires rest and hydration	Needs medical evaluation, and may require antibiotics
Needs antihistamines or allergy control measures	Don't overuse antibiotics, as they won't help here	Delays in treatment may lead to sinus complications

Sinus Health and Post-Nasal Drip

Post-nasal drip is often misdiagnosed or ignored until it causes chronic coughs, throat irritation or even ear issues in some cases. It may signal:

- **Chronic sinusitis** (with mucus constantly dripping into your throat)
- **Allergies** (creating excess clear mucus and often unresponsive to cold medications)
- **Silent reflux (GERD)** (where stomach acid irritates the nasal and throat linings)

- **Medication side effects** (especially from antihistamines or blood pressure drugs)

Left untreated, post-nasal drip may disturb sleep, inflame vocal cords or mimic asthma. Diagnosis often requires imaging or specialist input.

Small Fluid, Mighty Function

Saliva is not just moisture in your mouth. It's a multifunctional, constantly active fluid that supports digestion, oral health, immunity and even diagnosis. Produced primarily by the salivary glands, this clear, enzyme-rich liquid performs dozens of subtle tasks each minute, from breaking down food to protecting teeth from decay.

The Many Hats of Saliva

Saliva begins acting the moment you even think about food. Its enzymes initiate digestion before food reaches the stomach, while its lubricating properties help you chew, taste and swallow comfortably. In clinical settings, saliva is increasingly used for non-invasive diagnostics, from hormone testing (like cortisol) to COVID-19 screening and early cancer detection.

Dry Mouth

Dry mouth is a red flag. Reduced saliva production, known as xerostomia, may result from:

- Dehydration
- Medications (antidepressants, antihistamines or chemotherapy)
- Autoimmune disorders (for example, Sjögren's syndrome)

- Nerve damage or salivary gland dysfunction
- Chronic mouth breathing or smoking

Chronic dry mouth deserves evaluation, especially if accompanied by burning sensations or a persistent sore throat. It may otherwise lead to difficulty in chewing and speaking, bad breath, mouth ulcers or accelerated tooth decay.

Blood in Saliva and Oral Hygiene Alarms

Noticing blood in your saliva, especially when brushing, flossing or waking up should not be ignored. Common causes include:

- Gingivitis or periodontitis (gum disease from poor oral hygiene)
- Trauma or ulcers (accidental biting, sharp food or ill-fitting dental work)
- Vitamin deficiencies (particularly vitamin C and K)
- Systemic diseases (such as clotting disorders or severe infections)

Occasional pink-tinged saliva may result from vigorous brushing too.

However, frequent or unexplained bleeding requires professional assessment to rule out advanced periodontal disease or, more rarely, malignancy.

The Ear's Protective Cast

Often overlooked or underestimated, earwax (or cerumen) is a waxy substance which is secreted by glands in the outer ear canal to maintain ear health. In addition to earwax, the presence of other ear fluids, especially drainage, can sometimes signal infections, injuries or deeper systemic conditions, with variations across age groups.

Types of Earwax

Earwax is not one-size-fits-all. It exists in two genetically determined types, each with distinct characteristics.[29]

Wet earwax	Moist and sticky	Most commonly found in people of African or European descent	Often has a stronger odour, and can be more visible
Dry earwax	Flaky and light-coloured	Most common in East Asian and Native American populations	Typically has less odour, and accumulates in smaller amounts

The type of earwax can even correlate with other biological traits. For instance, people with wet earwax are more likely to produce underarm odour.

While normal earwax is self-cleaning, helping trap dust, debris and microorganisms, excess buildup can sometimes lead to symptoms like ear fullness, hearing difficulty or dizziness. Moreover, aggressive cleaning, especially with cotton swabs, can sometimes push wax deeper and cause impaction or injury.

Follow the Drainage

When the ear secretes fluid beyond wax, it is typically a red flag.

---

[29]Yoshiura, Kazuo, Akira Kinoshita, Takafumi Ishida, et al., 'A SNP in the *ABCC11* Gene Is the Determinant of Human Earwax Type', *Nature Genetics*, Vol. 38, No. 3, 2006, pp. 324–30, https://doi.org/10.1038/ng1733. Accessed on 8 December 2025.

Clear fluid	Occasionally, clear drainage may appear, and in rare cases, it could indicate cerebrospinal fluid following a head injury. Early detection allows timely medical care.
Cloudy/yellow fluid	Often a sign of a middle-ear infection. It usually responds well to treatment.
Bloody discharge	Can result from minor trauma, infection or a ruptured eardrum, and proper evaluation typically leads to effective management.
Foul-smelling pus	Suggests a chronic or bacterial infection, which can be addressed with appropriate medical attention.

Prompt evaluation is essential, especially when accompanied by pain, fever or hearing loss.

Ear Fluids across Age Groups

The source, cause and concern level of ear discharge can vary significantly by age.

In Children	*In Adults*	*In the Elderly*
Very common due to horizontal Eustachian tubes	More often associated with swimmer's ear (otitis externa), eczema of the ear canal, or the use of hearing aids or earbuds that trap moisture	Thinner skin and reduced earwax production may lead to dry, itchy ears

In Children	*In Adults*	*In the Elderly*
Fluid buildup can sometimes affect hearing or language development	Underlying systemic issues (like diabetes) may impair healing	Hearing aids and reduced mobility increase the risk of wax impaction and infection
Paediatric care is essential to prevent recurrent infections	Temporary irritation or minor infections are common and usually resolve quickly with proper hygiene and care	Drainage should always be evaluated, as symptoms may be subtler

Whether it's in a toddler with a fever or an elderly adult with subtle discharge, understanding ear fluids can mean the difference between a quick recovery and long-term hearing loss in some cases. Listen closely.

Nature's Lubricants

Understanding Different Types of Sweat

Sweat is essential, but not all sweat is the same. Therefore, understanding which type is flowing and why is crucial.

Type of Sweat	*Where It Appears*	*Triggers*	*What It May Be Telling You*
Eccrine	All over the body, especially, palms, soles and forehead	Heat, exertion and stress	May indicate overheating, hyperthyroidism or anxiety

Type of Sweat	*Where It Appears*	*Triggers*	*What It May Be Telling You*
Apocrine	Armpits, groin and nipples	Emotional stress and hormonal activity	Often associated with puberty, menopause, infections or shifts in body odour

Sometimes your body may suddenly sweat more than usual, especially at night or for no apparent reason. While it's often harmless, it can occasionally signal an underlying infection, like tuberculosis or a hormonal imbalance, such as hyperthyroidism. Paying attention early helps ensure prompt evaluation and care.

Body Odour and Bacterial Conversations

When body odour changes suddenly by becoming more pungent, sour or metallic, it often reflects changes in your microbial ecosystem or metabolic state.

Stress or anxiety	Heightened apocrine activity, signalling psychological or endocrine stress
New medications	May cause metabolic changes, sometimes indicating that the liver or kidneys are processing differently
Dietary changes	Foods high in sulphur, red meat or alcohol can influence body odour and place extra demand on detoxification systems

Persistent or foul odour may be the body's distress signal and point towards infections, metabolic imbalances or even certain cancers. Never mask it. Decode it.

Oily Skin, Acne and Hormonal Imbalances

Sebum helps your skin stay supple, but too much sebum can often lead to clogged pores, inflammation or breakouts. While commonly seen as a teenage issue, adult acne and excessive oil are also linked to hormonal imbalances, insulin resistance or even PCOS.

Persistent oily skin	May reflect elevated androgens or stress-related cortisol changes
Sudden acne flare-up	Can be linked to PCOS, thyroid imbalance or a reaction to medication
Dry skin patches	Sometimes associated with autoimmune conditions, eczema or nutritional deficiencies

Oily skin that won't respond to standard skincare may be your endocrine system seeking attention.

Phlegm Is the Reporter of Respiratory Health

When irritation, infection, or chronic damage strikes, the body responds with one of its most visible and audible defence mechanisms, that is, coughing and phlegm production. Whether triggered by pollution, pathogens or chronic inflammation, phlegm speaks volumes about lung health.

Productive vs Dry Cough

Understanding the type of cough is a critical first step in assessing your respiratory status.

Type of Cough	Presence of Phlegm?	Possible Causes	Clinical Significance
Dry cough	No	Viral infections, asthma, allergies, GERD or COVID-19	Usually reflects irritation or inflammation without mucus. Is often persistent but manageable with care.
Productive cough	Yes	Bacterial infections, chronic bronchitis or pneumonia	The body is actively clearing mucus that contains pathogens or debris, supporting the healing process.

A persistent dry cough may indicate inflammation, nerve irritation or early-stage viral infection, while a wet, phlegmy cough can point to infectious or chronic conditions that demand attention.

The Colour of Phlegm

Your phlegm's colour and texture are not incidental. They are reflective of the immune system's communication with the lungs.

Clear phlegm is generally normal, though it may also appear with mild irritation or allergies. White or grey phlegm can suggest a viral infection or chronic bronchitis, especially if it lingers. Yellow phlegm reflects an active immune response to an infection, while green usually points to a bacterial cause, such as bronchitis or pneumonia, and deserves medical attention. Brown phlegm may appear in smokers or those exposed to pollution, sometimes carrying traces of old blood. Red or pink phlegm indicates the presence of fresh blood and should always be taken seriously, as it can point to infections or, in rare cases, cancer. Black phlegm, though uncommon, may result from heavy pollution, fungal infection or coal dust exposure and it requires specialist care.

Changes in colour, amount or consistency of phlegm should never be ignored, especially if accompanied by fever, breathlessness or chest pain.

Smoking, Pollution and Chronic Lung Alarms

When the lungs are regularly exposed to cigarette smoke, polluted air or industrial chemicals, their natural defence system struggles to keep up. To protect themselves, the lungs produce excess mucus to trap harmful particles, but this often leads to constant congestion. At the same time, the tiny cilia (hair-like structures that normally sweep mucus out) can become damaged, making it harder to clear the airways. Over time, the irritation may even fuel chronic inflammation, which may change the structure of the lungs themselves.

These changes raise the risk of chronic bronchitis, emphysema and lung cancer. Even second-hand smoke and everyday urban air pollution can cause phlegm-related breathing problems, particularly in children and older adults, whose lungs are more vulnerable.

Chronic Respiratory Illnesses

When phlegm becomes a daily feature, the possibility of a chronic condition must be considered.

Bronchitis

- Characterized by a persistent cough with mucus
- Can be acute (infection-based) or chronic (long-term irritant exposure)
- Often worsens in winter or in polluted environments

COPD (Chronic Obstructive Pulmonary Disease)

- A progressive disease involving chronic bronchitis and emphysema
- Chronic productive cough, breathlessness and frequent infections are some of the symptoms
- Strongly linked to smoking history, but also seen in non-smokers exposed to pollution

Asthma and Cystic Fibrosis

- Involves overactive mucus glands
- Requires tailored management based on mucus consistency and reactivity

Takeaway: Every time you cough up phlegm, whether the message is mild irritation or chronic lung disease depends on what the mucus looks like, how often it appears and what else it brings along. In a world of increasing pollution and respiratory threats, learning to interpret these signals is essential.

The Stomach's Second Thoughts

Vomiting is never subtle. It is violent, raw and terrifyingly primal. It's your body saying, 'Something is wrong. Get it out.'

Colours, Contents and What They Mean

The colour, smell and texture of your vomit matter—sometimes, they mean everything.

What You See	*What It Might Mean*	*When to Worry*
Clear or white foam	Often due to an empty stomach or mild nausea	Usually harmless. Focus on rest and fluids
Yellow or green (bile)	May reflect intestinal backup, prolonged vomiting or gallbladder irritation	See a doctor if it continues or worsens
Bright red blood	Can result from tearing caused by violent retching or from bleeding ulcers	Get medical help right away
Black or coffee-ground-like	Indicates digested blood and is often linked to internal bleeding	Treat as an emergency. Go to the hospital immediately
Food that won't digest	May signal gastroparesis, obstruction or stomach motility issues	Concerning if frequent. A medical review is recommended
Foul-smelling or faecal	Suggests a serious intestinal blockage. It is often a late-stage problem	Life-threatening without prompt treatment

When you vomit and it doesn't feel normal, whether from intensity, frequency or what you see in the sink, that's when you need to pay attention.

Stool as the Gut's Daily Update

If you are not looking in the toilet bowl, you are ignoring one of your body's most consistent and honest alarms.

What Should Stool Look Like?

Healthy stool is:

- Medium to dark brown (due to bile)
- Well-formed, soft and sausage-shaped
- Passed easily and regularly (anywhere from three times a day to three times a week)

Deviations from this are often concerning body alarms.

What the Colour, Shape and Smell of Your Stool Reveal

Pale or clay-coloured stool	May signal a blocked bile duct or liver-related issue. It's worth checking promptly
Black, tarry stool	Can indicate bleeding in the stomach or upper gut, such as from ulcers. An urgent review is needed
Bright red stool	Often linked to haemorrhoids, anal fissures or bleeding lower in the intestines
Green stool	Could be from rapid digestion, bile changes or eating lots of greens. It is usually harmless
Yellow, greasy or floating stool	May reflect fat absorption problems, such as coeliac disease or pancreatitis
Loose or watery stool	Common with infections, food intolerances, IBS or even stress and anxiety
Hard, pellet-like stool	Typically, a sign of constipation or dehydration. Hydration and fibre could help

Ribbon-thin stool	Could point to narrowing from an obstruction or colorectal tumour. Needs a medical review
Extremely foul-smelling stool	May be due to infection, poor digestion or gut microbiome imbalance

Patterns That Demand Attention

- Sudden change in bowel habits
- Persistent diarrhoea or constipation
- Unexplained weight loss or fatigue
- Blood, mucus or oil in the stool
- Feeling of incomplete evacuation

Stool across the Lifespan

Children: Bright yellow or green stools are normal in infants. However, persistent diarrhoea and presence of mucus or blood in stools demands paediatric evaluation. Watch for signs of dehydration and food allergies.

Adults: Constipation or IBS-like patterns often point to lifestyle, diet or stress. Any bleeding, change in colour or pain should trigger a check-up.

Elderly: Constipation and faecal impaction are common, especially with medications. The presence of blood, pencil-thin stool or sudden changes can sometimes signal colorectal cancer or diverticulitis.

Tip: Look. Notice. Log. And never ignore what your stool is trying to say.

Why Do Doctors Care So Much about Urine?

Long before the advent of laboratory tests, healers and physicians used to observe the colour, smell and flow of urine. Even today, modern medicine regards urine as one of the most revealing and accessible diagnostic tools. From hydration to infection and from hormones to organ function, urine offers continuous updates on your internal environment.

Frequency, Colour, Smell and Clarity

Most people flush without a glance. That's a mistake, as every characteristic of your urine holds a clue.

Clear to pale yellow urine	A good sign of healthy hydration and well-functioning kidneys
Dark yellow/amber urine	Often due to dehydration, as the kidneys concentrate waste
Orange urine	Can signal liver or bile duct issues, or sometimes be a side effect of medication
Pink or red urine	May indicate blood in the urine (linked to infection, kidney stones or more serious causes like cancer)
Brown or cola-coloured urine	Could reflect advanced liver disease, muscle breakdown (rhabdomyolysis) or older internal bleeding
Cloudy urine	Commonly points to a urinary tract infection (UTI), especially if accompanied by burning or urgency
Foul-smelling urine	Often tied to bacterial infections or certain metabolic conditions

Sweet/fruity odour in urine	A red flag for uncontrolled diabetes and possible ketoacidosis. An urgent medical review is needed

If your urine colour changes suddenly or consistently, don't wait it out. Investigate.

Too little urine? Sometimes, it simply reflects dehydration, but it can also signal that the kidneys or fluid balance need closer attention. If it continues, it's best to check with a doctor.

UTI Symptoms Aren't Universal

Women	More prone to UTIs because of shorter urethras. Common signs include burning, urgency and pelvic discomfort
Men	Less frequent but often more complicated. A UTI may point to prostate involvement or sometimes an STI
Children	Symptoms may be subtle. So look for fever, tiredness, irritability or new episodes of bedwetting
Elderly	Confusion or sudden behavioural changes may be the only sign. Infections can be missed and may progress quickly, so pay attention

If confusion suddenly sets in in an older adult, rule out a UTI immediately.

Also, don't second-guess if you experience:

- Blood in your urine
- Pain or burning during urination
- Fever, chills or back pain
- Sweet or chemical-like smell
- Foamy urine or dramatically reduced output

The sooner you notice changes, the sooner you can take steps to protect your health.

What Every Woman Should Know

The colour, flow and texture of your menstrual blood provide valuable information about reproductive health and overall well-being. Paying attention to these patterns can help you understand your body and recognize changes that may need medical attention.

Bright red menstrual blood	This is fresh blood, and is usually normal and healthy
Dark brown or black menstrual blood	This is older blood, which is commonly seen at the start or end of a period
Watery and light menstrual blood	May indicate a vitamin or mineral deficiency or hormonal imbalance
Thick with clots (>1 inch)	Could be a sign of high oestrogen levels or uterine fibroids. A doctor's check-up is recommended if it continues
Pink or pale menstrual blood	Might suggest low oestrogen, anaemia, or the transition into perimenopause

Sudden or persistent changes in flow or colour should prompt medical consultation, especially if accompanied by fatigue, dizziness or irregular cycles.

Clots, Spotting and Bleeding between Periods

Not all bleeding follows a regular monthly schedule. Such variations can be harmless or may serve as early warning signs of underlying health issues.

Spotting mid-cycle	Light bleeding around ovulation is often normal, but it can also reflect temporary hormonal changes
Breakthrough bleeding	Common when using hormonal contraceptives, yet persistent bleeding may signal issues with the endometrium or cervix. Medical evaluation is advised if it continues
Large or frequent clots	May indicate uterine polyps, fibroids or, in some cases, early miscarriage. A doctor's assessment is recommended if this occurs
Bleeding after intercourse	It should never be ignored, as it could be a sign of infection, cervical erosion or, rarely, cervical cancer. Prompt medical attention is important

Menstruation is your body's monthly status report. Track it. Trust it. Talk about it.

'Could This Vaginal Discharge Be a Sign of Infection?'

In a world where silence around women's health persists, vaginal discharge still remains one of the most misunderstood and underestimated indicators of well-being.

Vaginal discharge is a natural part of the body, and it's not something to be ashamed of. Paying attention to its changes can help prevent infections, support fertility and allow early detection of potential health issues.

Understanding the Norm

Normal vaginal discharge changes throughout the menstrual cycle. It is produced by glands in the cervix and vagina to keep the area clean and maintain a protective acidic environment.

Phase	*Cervical Mucus Appearance*	*What It Means*
Post-menstrual (Days 1–5)	Dry or minimal	Oestrogen is low and the uterine lining has just been shed. Fertility is minimal
Pre-ovulation (Days 6–10)	Sticky or creamy white	Oestrogen starts rising. Fertility begins to increase as the body prepares for ovulation
Ovulation (Days 11–14)	Clear and stretchy like raw egg white	Peak fertility. Cervical mucus is designed to help sperm reach the egg
Post-ovulation (Days 15–28)	Thick, cloudy and reduced in volume	Progesterone rises. Fertility decreases and cervical mucus becomes thicker, making it harder for sperm to pass

A sudden deviation in volume, texture or odour outside this rhythm deserves attention.

When Discharge Signals Distress

Grey, fishy-smelling discharge	Often caused by bacterial vaginosis and is a common vaginal bacterial imbalance
Thick, white cottage cheese-like discharge	Usually indicates a fungal infection (Candida), commonly called a yeast infection
Yellow or green foul-smelling discharge	May signal trichomoniasis or other sexually transmitted infections (STIs). Medical consultation is recommended
Brown discharge	Typically, old blood from a recent period or early pregnancy (implantation)
Watery, persistent discharge	Could be due to cervical erosion or, rarely, cervical cancer. Medical evaluation is advised

If itching, burning, swelling or pain accompanies the discharge, seek medical evaluation immediately. Abnormal discharge should never be normalized or ignored.

What Every Man Should Know

Think of semen as a complex biological signal. Although often overlooked or awkward to discuss in cultural conversations, its composition, texture and timing of release can provide valuable insights into male reproductive health.

What Is Semen, Really?

Semen is a fluid primarily designed for reproduction, but it also acts as a barometer of male urogenital health. Its components come from multiple glands.

Healthy semen is typically white or slightly grey, with a jelly-like texture that liquefies in under thirty minutes.

When Discharge Occurs outside of Ejaculation

Not all semen-related discharge is sexual. Unexpected or spontaneous fluid may be body alarms.

Pre-ejaculate	A normal fluid released during sexual arousal. It helps lubricate the urethra and neutralize acidity to support sperm
Post-urination dribble	Common, especially with age or after intercourse, and usually harmless. It happens when small amounts of urine remain in the urethra
Clear or whitish urethral discharge at rest	May indicate an underlying condition such as urethritis, prostatitis or a sexually transmitted infection. Medical evaluation is recommended
Milky discharge during bowel movements	Could be a sign of ejaculatory duct obstruction or prostate inflammation. Seek medical advice if persistent or accompanied by other symptoms

Persistent or unusual discharge, particularly if foul-smelling, should be evaluated by a healthcare professional. Early attention can prevent complications and help maintain reproductive health.

Understanding Prostate Changes through Semen

The prostate plays a vital role in semen production. When it is inflamed or impaired, semen can change dramatically.

Blood in semen (Haematospermia)	May result from prostatitis, injury to the seminal vesicles or, rarely, prostate or seminal tract cancer. Evaluation by a healthcare professional is recommended
Yellow or green tint	Often indicates a bacterial or sexually transmitted infection. Medical assessment can confirm the cause
Painful ejaculation	Can be caused by prostatitis, urethritis or pelvic nerve issues. Seeking medical advice helps address discomfort and underlying conditions
Low semen volume	Commonly linked to ageing, hormonal changes, blockages in the reproductive tract, or dehydration. Lifestyle adjustments or medical consultation may help
No semen during climax	May occur due to retrograde ejaculation or as a side effect of prostate surgery. Evaluation can determine the cause and possible solutions

Men over fifty should pay attention to changes in semen, urinary flow and sexual function, as these may signal early signs of benign prostatic hyperplasia (BPH) or prostate health issues.

Early awareness allows better management.

The Hormone-Fertility Connection

Lifestyle and health factors such as stress, obesity or alcohol consumption can influence semen quality. Changes like low semen volume or watery texture may signal low testosterone, ductal obstruction or testicular dysfunction. Even in young, healthy men, monitoring semen changes after illness, medications or lifestyle shifts can help detect early imbalances and support reproductive health.

So, whether you are twenty-five or sixty-five, don't brush off subtle changes in texture, colour, frequency or sensation because in matters of fertility and function, time is an issue.

Observing Is an Art That Most People Ignore…

Consider Doraemon, the iconic robotic cat, admired not only for his gadgets but also for his vigilance. He always noticed subtle signs and acted early, thereby preventing problems before they grew. Your relationship with your body's fluids demands the same attentiveness.

Your bodily fluids often signal what is yet to surface in pain or visible symptoms. Thus, they offer a vital window for timely action.

What matters is awareness, attentiveness and respect for your body's messages. Like Doraemon, your insight mainly lies in observing the body alarms that are neither random nor trivial.

PART 4

PILLARS OF PREVENTIVE HEALTHCARE

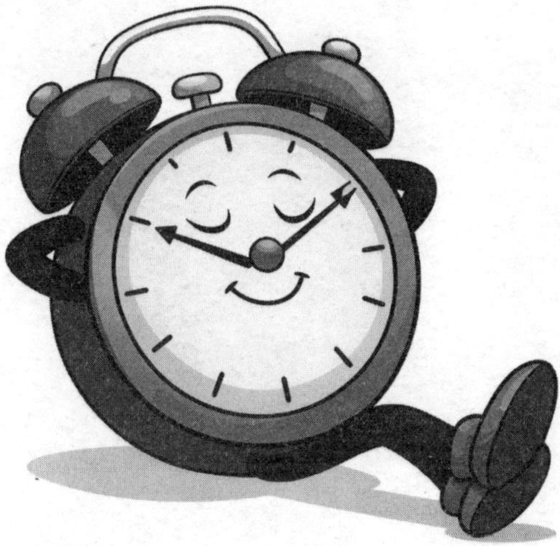

The Feel of a Healthy Body

Scientifically, we use virtually 100 per cent of our brain, just not all at once. Functional MRI scans show that even during sleep or simple tasks, multiple brain regions are active. The '10 per cent myth' likely originated from misinterpretations of early neurological research.

Every part of the brain has a known function (from regulating heart rate to enabling abstract thought or creativity). And its peak efficiency comes from a body in steady health.[30]

For much of this book, we have listened to the body's urgent alarms. We have delved deep into early symptom recognition and preclinical intervention, which is the essence of secondary prevention, because catching problems before they become serious is where true health mastery begins. While the world advocates for vaccination, diet and exercise, this book argues that health is also saved in the delicate window right after the first warning signs appear.

Now, it's time to turn the spotlight away from what is alarming and shine it on what sustains us.

So, what does a healthy body feel like?

The answer is deceptively simple and revolutionary in

[30]Boyd, Robynne, 'Do People Only Use 10 Percent of Their Brains?', *Scientific American*, 7 February 2008, https://tinyurl.com/3psnp5ed. Accessed on 8 December 2025.

its subtlety. A healthy body hums with effortless balance. It digests without complaint, breathes without thought, sleeps soundly without struggle, and moves fluidly without pain. It supports a mind that is sharp, a mood that is steady, and an energy that feels natural instead of forced.

This silence of well-being, which is often taken for granted, is the body's greatest gift to us.

This chapter invites you to discover that feeling of strength, to separate fact from fiction and to embrace a new definition of normal that celebrates the absence of alarm and the presence of harmony. It's because real health is about recognizing the beauty of what is working, just as much as it is about fixing what is broken. And in that recognition lies the realization that it is not enough to have a long life but to have one that is freer, more vibrant and healthier.

The Four Pillars of Secondary Prevention

You might think prevention begins and ends with vaccinations, diet or exercise, but there is also a deeper, more nuanced layer where your true power lies—secondary prevention. That is, the moment when you learn to read your body's subtle signals, act early and keep minor issues from escalating into major problems.

Stated below are the four essential pillars of secondary prevention that empower you to take control of your health before any illness takes hold.

Symptom Literacy

Developing symptom literacy means learning to recognize those early, often overlooked changes, such as a fleeting rash, a slight change in energy, or a subtle shift in sleep patterns.

Countless individuals have detected issues early simply by tuning in to these faint cues,[31] and you can too.

Timely Diagnostics

Knowing when to check and what to track transforms your actions in regard to health from reactive to proactive.

Think of routine screenings as your personal health GPS, which helps you navigate early warning signs. By keeping a simple health dashboard to track blood pressure, sleep quality, skin tone or nail condition, you create a baseline. This baseline helps you spot meaningful changes, and strategic investments in blood tests, imaging or hormonal panels further provide vital insights before symptoms surface.

This way, you are not guessing but monitoring intelligently.

Preclinical Intervention

What do you do when you feel 'off' but not sick?

This is the golden zone for intervention. Before medication, focus on foundational habits such as optimizing sleep, maintaining hydration, managing stress or considering targeted supplements. Small, timely changes here can often reverse trajectories and prevent full-blown illness.

Imagine someone who caught a creeping imbalance early,

---

[31]Lee, Jeehye, and Dong-Hee Ryu, 'Recognition of Early Cardiovascular Disease Symptoms in Hypertensive and Dyslipidemic Individuals of Icheon, Korea: Insights into Educational Levels and Health Literacy', *Healthcare (Basel)*, Vol. 12, No. 7, 2024, p. 736, https://doi.org/10.3390/healthcare12070736; Ansari, Arshi, Monika Agarwal, Vijay K. Singh, Kumari Nutan, Suajata Deo, and Trideep Jyoti Deori, 'Breast Cancer Literacy: Status of Peripheral Health Workers in Lucknow', *Asian Pacific Journal of Cancer Care*, Vol. 8, No. 2, 2023, pp. 287–94, https://doi.org/10.31557/apjcc.2023.8.2.287-294. Both accessed on 8 December 2025.

adjusted lifestyle factors and avoided years of chronic disease. That's the power of preclinical action.

Health Identity and Personal Agency

Finally, your health journey is uniquely yours.

Base your approach on awareness, rather than on fear and worry. Partner with your healthcare providers with knowledge and confidence, rather than waiting passively. Adopt a proactive, mindful approach to healthcare every day.

Once you embrace this sense of agency, prevention stops being an emergency measure and becomes part of everyday life.

Health Often Feels like Nothing at All

By now, you might be expecting the usual clichés that 'a healthy body glows,' 'you feel energized,' and 'listen to your gut.' However, this is not that section. This is not a motivational listicle. This is a clinical, grounded reminder of what physiological normalcy looks and feels like. After chapters of decoding what can go wrong, it's time to honour what it feels like when everything is invisibly right.

It's about knowing with calm confidence that your systems are in sync.

Because in a world obsessed with symptoms, scans and supplements, we have lost touch with a profound truth: Health often feels like nothing at all.

Let's break down what that 'nothing' looks like scientifically, sensibly and reassuringly.

'I Don't Chase Sleep...'

Sleep quality is not measured by how long you are in bed,

but by how efficiently your body uses that time.

- You fall asleep within ten to twenty minutes (which is a sign of good melatonin release and minimal sleep resistance).
- You wake zero to one times per night, without full arousal or struggle to return to sleep.
- You wake up refreshed, with no muscle soreness, jaw tension or mental fog.
- Dream recall is occasional, not constant. Your brain cycles through REM and non-REM efficiently.

'My Body Doesn't Remind Me to Breathe...'

Your cardiopulmonary system speaks loudest when it is struggling. When it is healthy, it's silent.

- You are unaware of your breathing and heartbeat at rest, and it means that your autonomic nervous system is well-regulated.
- After light exertion (for example, one flight of stairs), your breathing normalizes within 30 to 60 seconds.
- There is no random chest tightness, skipped beats or need to sigh frequently.

'My Gut Isn't the Centre of My Day...'

A healthy gut is not attention-seeking.

- You feel genuine hunger before meals and natural satiety without heaviness.
- Bowel movements are regular (daily or every other day), formed and easy to pass.
- Occasional gas or burping is normal. It reflects gut flora at work.

- You are unaware of your stomach and intestines most of the day and that's a good sign.

'The Glow of Health Is Subtle...'

The skin is the largest organ and a reliable biomarker of internal balance.

- Your skin feels comfortable (not tight, flaky, itchy or burning without cause).
- Hair fall of up to hundred strands a day is physiologically normal and fluctuates with seasons, stress or age.
- Nails grow steadily (one to three mm per month) and remain free of ridges, pitting or unnatural colour changes.
- Minor bruises heal in under a week, reflecting normal capillary function and clotting.

'Fatigue Knows Its Limits...'

Forget the artificial 'high.' Think sustained readiness.

- You wake up with enough energy to begin your day without stimulants.
- A mild midday dip is natural. Crashing, however, is not.
- You can think, speak and perform daily tasks without needing sugar, caffeine or naps to get through.
- Post-meal energy dips are brief and tolerable. Your insulin response is on track.

'Focus Comes without Force...'

Mental wellness is deeply intertwined with systemic health.

- Your mood is stable (with fluctuations that match life events).

- You experience mental clarity, especially during familiar or routine tasks.
- You are not frequently forgetful, emotionally volatile or apathetic without a clear cause.
- You can concentrate for thirty to ninety minutes at a time (which is standard attention span in healthy adults).

'Stiffness Is a Stranger...'

Joint mobility is a measure of wellness. The easier the motion, the healthier the body.

- You sit, stand and walk without pain or hesitation.
- Minor joint popping or cracking is common and benign if it's not painful or associated with swelling.
- You are unaware of your posture most of the time, meaning that your muscles are supporting you efficiently.
- You wake up without morning stiffness that lasts longer than a few minutes.

'I Feel Neither Too Hot Nor Too Cold...'

Even subtler signs matter.

- You rarely feel too hot or too cold without an environmental cause. This means that your thermoregulation is stable.
- You don't frequently fall sick. Less than two to three mild infections a year is average for most healthy adults.
- Menstrual cycles (if applicable) are predictable and tolerable, and libido is stable, reflecting hormonal balance.

In truth, a healthy body doesn't constantly announce itself. It doesn't feel like a 'buzz' or a 'glow.' It just feels like not having to think about your body all the time.

Mind you, this isn't anticlimactic.

This is profound. Because when you understand what's right, you become a better judge of what's not.

What's Normal, Even When It Feels Strange

Your body constantly communicates through subtle signs that may often be misunderstood as warnings but are, in fact, perfectly normal variations. For instance, a black or brownish discolouration on the tongue, commonly referred to as 'black hairy tongue,' occurs due to harmless accumulation of dead skin cells or bacteria and is frequently influenced by factors such as smoking or recent antibiotic use. Similarly, a white coating on the tongue upon waking is usually a result of mild dehydration or transient fungal presence, and it typically resolves with adequate hydration or oral hygiene.

The appearance of new moles or freckles during adolescence and adulthood (particularly after sun exposure) is generally benign as well. These moles tend to be symmetrical, uniform in colour and stable over time. Also, eye-related phenomena like frequent blinking and occasional eyelid twitching are natural reflexes which are often triggered by fatigue, stress or dryness and usually require no intervention. In the realm of digestion, passing gas, experiencing mild bloating or occasional burping after meals reflects normal gastrointestinal function, while variations in bowel movement frequency within a reasonable range are commonly expected.

Minor muscle twitching or cramps, especially following physical exertion or periods of stress, are common too and they seldom indicate serious pathology. Joint cracking sounds arise from the release of gas bubbles within synovial fluid and don't always signify cartilage damage. Further, fluctuations in energy, such as brief mid-afternoon slumps, align with circadian rhythms and don't inherently denote illness. Also, nails may develop vertical ridges or mild peeling as part of natural ageing or minor nutritional changes without signalling disease.

Increased frequency of urination associated with high fluid or caffeine intake is normal too and should be interpreted in context. Likewise, occasional menstrual spotting between cycles often results from hormonal shifts or transient stress and is rarely a cause for alarm.

Mild night sweats or increased sweating in warm environments are also physiological mechanisms (for thermoregulation), most of the time.

Sexual health has its spectrum of normalcy as well. Variations in libido, ranging from fluctuating desire to periods of low interest, can reflect natural hormonal cycles, stress levels or emotional states and are not inherently pathological. Occasional changes in sexual function or response often correspond with lifestyle factors and don't always require medical intervention unless persistent.

Emotional fluctuations such as occasional mood swings, mild anxiety during stressful periods or transient difficulty concentrating are also part of the normal human experience. These don't necessarily indicate psychiatric illness but rather the dynamic nature of brain chemistry adapting to internal and external stimuli.

Understanding such normal bodily signs across physical, sexual and mental domains is extremely crucial in developing a refined awareness that distinguishes routine variations from genuine health concerns. This discernment empowers you to approach your well-being with confidence and supports the proactive ethos of secondary prevention.

Health Myths and Misconceptions We Have All Heard

When it comes to health, advice often comes wrapped in myths and half-truths. It is passed down through families, reinforced by culture or repeated so often that they feel like facts.

Now, let's take a closer look at some of the most common health myths and misconceptions, keeping in mind that what we call a 'myth' is not always so straightforward or consistent.

'Don't Stand while Drinking Water'

You might have heard that gulping water while standing is somehow harmful and that it's better to sit down or even lie back to let the water 'properly absorb' or to protect your kidneys. This belief is surprisingly widespread and is passed down through generations as common wisdom. However, does it hold up under scientific scrutiny?

The truth is, your body is remarkably efficient at managing hydration, no matter your posture. Water absorption primarily happens in the small intestine, and gravity or body position plays an insignificant role in this process. Your kidneys are also the master regulators of your fluid balance and work continuously to maintain homeostasis, adjusting urine concentration and volume regardless of whether you are sitting, standing or lying down.[32]

---

[32]Jones, Karen L., Deirdre O'Donovan, Michael Horowitz, Antonietta Russo, Yong Lei, and Trygve Hausken, 'Effects of Posture on Gastric Emptying, Transpyloric Flow, and Hunger after a Glucose Drink in Healthy Humans', *Digestive Diseases and Sciences*, Vol. 51, No. 8, 2006, pp. 1331–38, https://doi.org/10.1007/s10620-005-9010-3. Accessed on 8 December 2025.

So, while sipping water calmly can aid mindful hydration, the idea that standing somehow impairs absorption or harms your kidneys is a myth. The real priority is simply to drink enough water throughout the day and stay hydrated.

'Don't Use a Pillow; It's Bad for Your Spine'

Many people believe that using a pillow can cause spinal misalignment or lead to chronic neck pain. Some even avoid pillows altogether or choose extremely flat ones, hoping to protect their necks from strain.

However, science tells a more nuanced story. The role of a pillow is actually to support your natural spinal alignment, which varies depending on how you sleep. Side sleepers typically need a firmer, thicker pillow to fill the gap between their head and shoulder, while back sleepers benefit from a medium-soft pillow to maintain the neck's natural curve. Stomach sleepers, though less common, often require very thin or no pillows (to avoid overextension).[33]

Choosing the right pillow height, firmness and material is essential to prevent neck discomfort and promote restorative sleep. Rather than avoiding pillows altogether, it's about finding the one that suits your unique anatomy and sleep position.

'Don't Shower on a Full Stomach'

A common belief is that showering immediately after a meal, especially with hot water, can disrupt digestion by diverting

---

[33]Chun-Yiu, J.P., Sharon Tsang Man-Ha, and Allan Fu Chak-Lun, 'The Effects of Pillow Designs on Neck Pain, Waking Symptoms, Neck Disability, Sleep Quality and Spinal Alignment in Adults: A Systematic Review and Meta-Analysis', *Clinical Biomechanics (Bristol)*, Vol. 85, 2021, https://doi.org/10.1016/j.clinbiomech.2021.105353. Accessed on 8 December 2025.

blood flow away from the stomach. The idea behind it is that blood is 'pulled' towards the skin to regulate temperature, leaving less available for digestive processes.

In reality, digestion does require increased blood flow to the gastrointestinal tract, but the body efficiently manages blood distribution to support multiple functions simultaneously. While hot showers do cause some blood vessels near the skin to dilate, this does not significantly reduce blood flow to the gut. The cardiovascular system often compensates to maintain adequate circulation.

Having said that, immediately engaging in vigorous activities like hot showers or intense exercise right after a heavy meal can indeed cause mild discomfort for some individuals. However, the evidence is limited on whether or not to shower on a full stomach.[34]

'Everyone Should Take Multivitamins'

Many people believe that taking daily multivitamins is necessary to fill nutritional gaps and maintain optimal health. The idea that supplements are a universal solution has become widespread and is often promoted as an easy way to prevent deficiencies.

However, evidence shows that while multivitamins are valuable for correcting specific nutrient deficiencies, they provide little to no benefit for well-nourished individuals consuming a balanced diet. In fact, excessive or unnecessary supplementation can sometimes lead to adverse effects, such as toxicity or nutrient imbalances.[35]

---

[34]Watson, Kathryn, 'Is It Bad to Bathe Shortly after Eating?', *Healthline*, 19 November 2020, https://tinyurl.com/yz2s7rba. Accessed on 8 December 2025.
[35]'Is There Really Any Benefit to Multivitamins?', *Johns Hopkins Medicine*, https://tinyurl.com/4xt4wbpb. Accessed on 8 December 2025.

The best strategy remains obtaining vitamins and minerals primarily from a varied or balanced diet rich in whole foods. Supplements should be tailored to individual needs, ideally under professional guidance.

'Detox Diets Flush out Toxins'

The wellness world is flooded with claims that certain diets, juices or supplements can 'flush out toxins' and reset your body, promoting rapid health improvements.

However, your body already has a highly effective detoxification system. Your liver, kidneys, lungs, skin and even your gut continuously work together to neutralize or eliminate toxins. These processes happen naturally, 24/7, without the need for restrictive diets or expensive cleanses.

There is no credible evidence anyway that detox diets enhance or accelerate this biological process. In fact, some detox plans can be nutritionally unbalanced or even harmful in the long term.[36] In short, your body is designed to detox itself. Supporting it with hydration, sleep, balanced nutrition and stress management is far more effective or safer than any marketed cleanse.

'Don't Hunch Too Close to the TV'

For generations, parents have warned children not to sit too close to the television, fearing it could damage their eyesight. The belief that proximity to screens causes long-term harm remains common.

However, science tells a different story here. Sitting close to a screen does not cause permanent eye damage, but it

[36]Kubala, Jillian, '"Detox Diets": Does Science Support the Claims?', *MedicalNewsToday*, 1 May 2021, https://tinyurl.com/y765jypb. Accessed on 8 December 2025.

can lead to temporary eye strain, also known as asthenopia. Symptoms may include tired eyes, headaches or blurred vision, especially after prolonged exposure, but these effects are reversible with rest and good visual hygiene.[37]

Thus, the real concern isn't distance but screen time duration, poor lighting and lack of breaks.

When 'Myths' Are True

Not all health myths deserve to be debunked. Some linger because they hold a sliver of truth that science eventually affirms. Take the old belief that you can catch a cold from being out in the cold. While viruses are the actual cause, studies now show that exposure to low temperatures can often suppress immune responses in the nasal passages, making you more susceptible to infection. So, while cold weather doesn't carry viruses, it does create the right conditions for them to thrive.[38]

Then, there is the classic carrot story that 'it is good for your eyes.' While no amount of carrots will give you night vision, they are rich in beta-carotene, which the body converts to vitamin A (a nutrient essential for maintaining good eyesight). Severe deficiency can sometimes cause real vision problems, including night blindness. In that sense, carrots really do help support ocular health.

And yes, the apple-a-day proverb isn't just rhyming advice.

---

[37] Bedinghaus, Troy, 'Optimizing TV Viewing Distances to Prevent Eye Fatigue', *verywell health*, 12 August 2025, https://tinyurl.com/c5zsyp29. Accessed on 8 December 2025.

[38] 'Scientists Uncover Biological Explanation behind Why Upper Respiratory Infections Are More Common in Colder Temperatures', Mass General Brigham, 6 December 2022, https://tinyurl.com/y2awsva3. Accessed on 8 December 2025.

Apples are packed with fibre, antioxidants and polyphenols that have been linked to a lower risk of heart disease, diabetes and certain cancers.[39] While no single fruit is a cure-all, this one comes close to representing how consistent, small dietary choices can shape your long-term health.

In a world where myths often mislead, it is refreshing to find that some of them were just early observations, intuitively passed down until science had the tools to explain why they worked.

Sometimes, it turns out, tradition did get it right.

Finally, the Frankenstein Metaphor

Consider a ship that has replaced all of its parts over time. Is it still the same vessel?

Health, too, is more than fixing broken pieces.

Mary Shelley's *Frankenstein* tells the story of a man who tried to create life by stitching together parts from different bodies. The resulting being moved in jerky, uncoordinated ways. It was alive, yet it struggled to function as a whole. Its challenge lay not only in its appearance but also in the lack of harmony within itself.

Our bodies are very different from Frankenstein's creation. We are not a collection of disconnected parts. Muscles, organs, nerves and cells constantly communicate, adapt and repair.

---

[39]Kim, Sun Jo, Nguyen Hoang Anh, Cheol Woon Jung, Nguyen Phuoc Long, Seongoh Park, Young Hyun Cho, Young Cheol Yoon, Eun Goo Lee, Mina Kim, Eui Young Son, Tae Ha Kim, Yingqian Deng, Johan Lim, and Sung Won Kwon, 'Metabolic and Cardiovascular Benefits of Apple and Apple-Derived Products: A Systematic Review and Meta-Analysis of Randomized Controlled Trials', *Frontiers in Nutrition*, Vol. 9, 2022, https://doi.org/10.3389/fnut.2022.766155. Accessed on 8 December 2025.

They work together continuously, even before we consciously notice any signs of imbalance or illness.

Unlike the disjointed creature of fiction, our bodies are on our side.

When we honour this partnership, life feels lighter, energy flows more freely, and health becomes a living experience that we can enjoy every day.

Acknowledgements

Writing *The Body Alarm* has been both a professional extension and a personal revelation for me. Years of medical practice have shown me how often we treat illness instead of understanding it—a tendency that strongly reflects the misplaced focus of our times. My gratitude goes to Mr Dibakar Ghosh, Editorial Director at Rupa Publications, whose thoughtful encouragement persuaded me to write on this subject. Having known my medical work for some time, he gave the book its first true form through his belief in the subject's relevance.

My heartfelt gratitude also goes to my parents: to my father, Ajay Gupta, whose life experiences with a preventable disability deepened my understanding and awareness; and to my mother, Deepshikha Gupta, who has always been my pillar of strength and closest friend. To my brother, Aakash, for his constant encouragement; to Dr Twinkle, for her guiding presence; and to my husband, Ishaan Gupta, for his steadfast love, patience and belief in me throughout this journey. To my family as a whole, thank you for being both my anchor and my inspiration.

I am also thankful to the patients, mentors, colleagues and thought leaders who, knowingly or unknowingly, contributed insights that shaped every chapter. Though too numerous to name, each has left a lasting imprint on this book. I am especially grateful to Jagriti Sharma, a valued member of my team, whose enthusiasm in engaging with my ongoing research has enriched this work.

Finally, to every reader seeking to understand their own body better, I thank you for your curiosity, and I hope *The Body Alarm* helps you embrace body literacy as your most powerful ally in health.